COST-EFFECTIVENESS ANALYSES IN HEALTH

COST-EFFECTIVENESS ANALYSES IN HEALTH

A Practical Approach

Second Edition

PETER MUENNIG

JB JOSSEY-BASS

Published by Jossey-Bass
A Wiley Imprint
989 Market Street, San Francisco, CA 94103-1741—www.josseybass.com

Jossey-Bass books and products are available through most bookstores. To contact Jossey-Bass directly call our Customer Care Department within the U.S. at 800-956-7739, outside the U.S. at 317-572-3986, or fax 317-572-4002.

Jossey-Bass also publishes its books in a variety of electronic formats. Some content that appears in print may not be available in electronic books.

Library of Congress Cataloging-in-Publication Data

Muennig, Peter.
    Cost-effectiveness analyses in health : a practical approach/Peter Muennig. — 2nd ed.
        p. ;   cm.
    Includes bibliographical references and index.
    ISBN-13: 978-0-7879-9556-0 (cloth)
        1. Medical care—United States—Cost effectiveness.   2. Medical care, Cost of—United States.   I. Title.
        [DNLM: 1. Cost-Benefit Analysis—methods.   2. Health Care Costs.   3. Quality of Life. W 74 M948c 2008]
    RA410.5.M84   2008
    338.4'33621—dc22

                                                                        2007026832

Printed in the United States of America
SECOND EDITION

HB Printing   10 9 8 7 6 5 4 3 2 1

CONTENTS

TABLES, FIGURES, & EXHIBITS

TABLES

FIGURES

EXHIBITS

PREFACE

Cost-effectiveness analysis is one of the fastest-growing fields in health research, but it has lacked an instruction manual until now. Other books address the theoretical aspects of cost-effectiveness analysis, but *Cost-Effectiveness Analyses in Health: A Practical Approach* teaches students how to perform cost-effectiveness research. The art of cost-effectiveness analysis is explored using real-world examples. In this book, you will learn how to find and evaluate data, build a simple decision analysis model, test the model, and present the results in a research paper. The only skills you will need to complete this book are basic math skills, though learning cost-effectiveness analysis will be easier for you if you have some spreadsheet skills and a basic knowledge of epidemiology and biostatistics.

Cost-Effectiveness Analyses in Health uses teaching techniques akin to the natural learning or immersion approach to language in which students learn a new language by speaking rather than studying grammar. In this book, problems are anticipated and solved in context, making the theory easy to appreciate and learn. The book can also be read without actually doing the examples, allowing for the study of theory without a practical component.

Public health students and professionals familiar with basic epidemiology and biostatistics research can skip the relevant supplemental chapters (Chapters Eleven and Twelve). However, this book also provides inexperienced students with a basic set of epidemiological and biostatistical tools relating to cost-effectiveness analysis.

Public health students, medical students, health economists, biomedical researchers, physicians, policymakers, and health managers should all find this book informative and fun. Since cost-effectiveness analysis is being used to evaluate medical interventions worldwide, the book uses approaches and examples that are applicable to both industrialized and developing countries. It teaches students how to evaluate interventions specific to infectious disease (a common type of analysis in developing countries) as well as chronic disease (a common type of analysis in developed countries). It also addresses issues specific to evaluating the cost-effectiveness of public health programs as well as problems specific to clinical medicine.

This book is written using a concise, structured format and has been tested in cost-effectiveness courses in the basic health science, medical school, and graduate school of public health settings. To use this book as a practical tool, students need a computer (and, optionally, a connection to the Internet). Web addresses to free spreadsheet software and decision analysis software are provided.

HOW TO USE THIS BOOK

In addition to introducing the core concepts of cost-effectiveness analysis, this book walks students through basic cost-effectiveness analyses. To fully benefit from the book, students should complete the exercises in each chapter; these exercises guide students through the process of obtaining electronic data, analyzing the medical literature, building a decision analysis tree, and conducting a sensitivity analysis.

Different students have different needs. The following points should help you make the most effective use of this book:

■ *Using this book for theoretical study alone.* Health managers and clinicians often wish to understand cost-effectiveness analysis methods but do not wish to conduct research. This book has been designed to allow students to understand the field of cost-effectiveness analysis using an applied approach. Still, the theory can be learned by simply following along without working on the examples in each chapter.

■ *Using this book as a textbook.* Instructors teaching courses that have biostatistics and epidemiology as prerequisites may skip Chapter Eleven; however, this chapter provides an excellent review of those concepts applicable to cost-effectiveness research. Introductory courses in cost-effectiveness analysis should skip Chapter Twelve, which is intended only for students who are actively working on a research project.

■ *Using this book for self-study.* Those who are actively working on a cost-effectiveness research question will find Chapter Twelve invaluable but might not need as much background information (found in Chapters One to Three) as beginning students.

■ *Using Internet resources.* This book provides links to data sources, journals, and other useful cost-effectiveness resources on the Internet. The Internet is a critical resource for cost-effectiveness research, but as we all know, the addresses for Web pages sometimes change. For this reason, links to specific Web pages are provided alongside links to the organizations that host these pages and are maintained at http://www.pceo.org/datasources.html.

A NOTE ON METHODS

In 1996, the U.S. Public Health Service's Panel on Cost-Effectiveness in Health and Medicine released methodological standards for conducting cost-effectiveness analyses. These standards were developed in response to a wide degree of variation in the ways in which such analyses were conducted. The use of disparate approaches to cost-effectiveness analysis sometimes leads to widely different study results when different research groups examine the cost-effectiveness of a single screening test or medical treatment.

For example, in the introduction to their book, the Panel on Cost-Effectiveness in Health and Medicine notes that the published cost-effectiveness of screening mammography for the detection of breast cancer varies from cost savings to $80,000 per quality-adjusted life-year gained (Gold, Siegel, Russell, and Weinstein, 1996).

To address problems with variation in the methods used from one study to the next, the Panel on Cost-Effectiveness in Health and Medicine developed a reference case analysis, which renders studies more comparable, easier to understand, and more useful to a broader array of consumers of cost-effectiveness data. Although the reference case standards were designed by the U.S. Public Health Service, the methods are applicable to cost-effectiveness analyses conducted in any country.

Cost-Effectiveness Analyses in Health adheres closely to the principles forwarded by this panel and was developed with some of its members. As the panel acknowledges, a reference case analysis is simply a set of standards. Well-conceived analyses that do not adhere to the reference case analysis are, of course, perfectly valid. The government or an insurance company may be interested in commissioning a study to answer a question that cannot be addressed within the framework of a reference case analysis. Nonetheless, since it was designed to apply to a broad array of professionals interested in the results of a cost-effectiveness analysis, the reference case analysis is comprehensive enough to provide students with all of the tools necessary to conduct any cost-effectiveness analyses. By building this book around the recommendations of the Panel on Cost-Effectiveness in Health and Medicine, I believe that this book will help students become leaders in the growing field of cost-effectiveness research.

ACKNOWLEDGMENTS

I would foremost like to thank my partner, Celina Su, the finder of lost objects. I also thank the countless students, contributors, reviewers, and mentors. Special thanks to Josh Zivin for his contributions to the lab manual, Sherry Glied for all of her support (including my reckless pursuit of academic projects like this book), Hala Al Saraf for diligence to editing in the face of adversity, Kamran Khan who started working with me as a student but ended up a teacher, Danny Pallin for being my perpetual mentor and dear friend, and all of my friends who put up with me when I am stressed out. Thanks, too, to all the readers who provided the feedback that made this major rewriting of the book possible.

THE AUTHOR

Peter Muennig is an assistant professor at Columbia University. He attended medical school at the University of California, San Diego and completed residency training at the New York City Department of Health/Columbia University Preventive Medicine Residency Program. Previously he directed the Program in Cost-Effectiveness and Outcomes at New School University, consulted for Health Canada and the Centers for Disease Control and Prevention, and was an assistant professor at the Sophie Davis School of Biomedical Education. He has published numerous studies in the medical literature and has won numerous awards for teaching. His research has changed health policies in various U.S. states and Canada. It has also influenced policy in the United Kingdom and Australia. His work has been discussed in the *New York Times,* CNN, Reuters, and numerous other media outlets.

Muennig's research explores methods for elucidating unforeseen solutions to vexing domestic and international health policy questions affecting socioeconomically disadvantaged populations. He primarily employs cost-effectiveness analyses with the intent of reducing socioeconomic disparities through more efficient use of societal resources in instances where the optimal decision is not intuitive. For example, he has explored the cost-effectiveness of approaches to reducing infectious disease in immigrant populations. More recently, his research has focused on education interventions as a means to improve health.

COST-EFFECTIVENESS ANALYSES IN HEALTH

CHAPTER

1

INTRODUCTION TO COST-EFFECTIVENESS

OVERVIEW

IMAGINE THAT you are the director of a large cancer society. Your day-to-day duties require you to conduct some research and oversee employees whose job is to compile data and make health recommendations. One morning you sit down with a cup of coffee and toast, and when you open the morning paper, you find that one of your society's recommendations—that women between the ages of forty and sixty receive screening mammography for breast cancer—has made the headline news: an elderly-rights group is suing your society. This group argues that your recommendation unfairly discriminates against the elderly because you have implied that women over the age of sixty should not be screened for breast cancer.

You rush to the office and find that the teams that made the recommendation are already in a heated meeting. They have split into two factions, and each group is now accusing the other of making bad decisions. But did they? You manage to calm everyone down and review the process they used to arrive at their recommendation. You learn that both groups were concerned that recommending mammograms for women over a wider age range might become very costly, thereby jeopardizing screening for women who might benefit from screening mammography the most.

One group argued that it made sense to screen older rather than younger women: mammography works better in older women, who have less dense breast tissue. Older women, they reasoned, were less likely to have a falsely positive mammogram and therefore would be less likely to suffer unnecessary procedures or surgery. Unnecessary interventions, they noted, place women at risk for surgical complications, are psychologically traumatic, are costly, and may do more harm than good.

The other group argued that it was unwise to actively screen all elderly women with mammography, because women who had breast cancer would die from other natural causes before the cancer had a chance to spread. After all, breast cancer can take over a decade to kill, and the life expectancy of older people is limited. Therefore, they reasoned, elderly women would be subjected to an uncomfortable and expensive screening test that would have little impact on the length of their lives. Besides, who would want to undergo chemotherapy in the precious remaining years of their lives?

Both factions made arguments based on sound scientific, economic, and social research, but which group was right? You and your employees decide to conduct a more extensive analysis of the costs and benefits of breast cancer screening and plan to send out a press release to this effect. But where do you start?

You might start by having a team estimate the likelihood that older women will die of breast cancer if they are not screened and have another team estimate the number of women who are likely to have false-positive mammograms at different ages. You might also wish to obtain information on the number of years of life that mammography will save, the quality of life for women who have different stages of breast cancer, and the psychological impact of a positive test result among women who do not in fact have breast cancer (**false-positive test results**). Because both teams were concerned about the costs of mammography, you may also wish to calculate the cost of screening mammography and the cost of all of the medical care that might be averted by detecting breast cancer at an early stage. Finally, because each team is interested in knowing whether women in both age groups might benefit from mammography, you decide that the costs and health benefits of screening each group should be compared to not screening women at all. If all of these factors were put together in a systematic manner, you would have conducted a cost-effectiveness analysis.

■ ■ ■

WHY COST-EFFECTIVENESS IS USEFUL

Now let's take a step back and consider why all of this is important in the first place. Certainly you want to know whether mammography is going to lead to net improvements or net declines in health. If it's only going to hurt people, we certainly don't want to do it. But if we know it helps, we also want to know whether it is affordable.

What does "affordable" mean when you are talking about human life? Take a moment to imagine what the society we live in could do with an infinite amount of money. We could build a huge public transportation system that eliminates car accidents, pollution, and noise. We could use only solar power and switch to 100 percent recycling, eliminating the major remaining causes of pollution; this would greatly reduce environmental carcinogens and oxidizing agents that cause cancer, heart disease, and premature aging. In addition, it would delay global warming, which threatens to put much of civilization under water, leading to countless deaths in the process. We could completely mechanize industry, eliminating occupational accidents. Finally, we could create a highly advanced health system that provides full MRI body scans and comprehensive laboratory screening tests for everyone in the population to ensure that cancers and other disorders are detected at the earliest possible stage.

As it is, there are very few nations that can even provide safe drinking water to all their citizens. The challenge, then, is to figure out how best to spend the money we have so that the quantity and quality of life can be maximized.

Thus, even if mammography screening for breast cancer is on the whole effective, it is conceivable that the money spent on it could save more lives if it went toward something else. Cost-effectiveness analysis helps determine how to maximize the quality and quantity of life in a particular society that is constrained by a particular budget.

We'll get deeper into this later in the book, but let's examine the specifics of the example to illustrate how resource allocation might work. Assume that the U.S. Congress decided to allocate $1 trillion to the competing health projects mentioned above. It could choose public transportation, greatly reducing pollution (a cause of pneumonia, cancer, and heart disease) and motor vehicle accidents (the fifth leading cause of death). It could invest in clean energy, reducing dependence on oil while reducing air pollution. Or it could choose the universal MRI strategy, detecting more tumor-producing cancers, some of which can be cured if detected early. If Congress knew the cost per year of life saved, it would know how to maximize the number of lives saved with the $1 trillion investment.

One thing that might strike some readers as a bit strange about this hypothetical situation is that we are essentially deciding who lives and who dies. If we save the mothers and fathers with cancerous tumors by opting for universal MRI examinations, many sons and daughters will die in car accidents as a result. Behind these numbers are real people affected by whatever decision is ultimately made. The more tangible the lives affected are, the more difficult the decision becomes.

As one famous physician, Paul Farmer (2004), points out, you cannot let a person die in front of you when you know that an effective treatment exists. Is the solution therefore to start a medical clinic, even if it comes at the expense of a more effective vaccination campaign? We might know that one intervention saves more lives than the other. However, when the most cost-effective intervention saves lives we will never see—lives that lie abstracted in numbers—it is more difficult to rationalize the choice.

Nevertheless, policymakers must often make abstracted decisions based on data from cost-effectiveness analysis, and these sometimes involve decisions that improve survival for one group at the cost survival for another. (We'll see an actual example of this later in the book.) These decisions become more abstract when quality-of-life issues are added to the mix of life-and-death issues.

ELEMENTS OF COST-EFFECTIVENESS ANALYSIS

Just as a driver really only needs to know about the accelerator, brake, and gearshift before driving a car for the first time, this section provides the basic parts of a cost-effectiveness analysis that you need to have in your head before you can start getting down to business.

Health Interventions

A **health intervention** can be a treatment, screening test, or primary prevention technique (for example, vaccinating children to prevent measles). Health interventions typically reduce the incidence rate of disease or its complications, improve the quality of life lived with disease, or improve life expectancy. Most produce some combination of these benefits. The benefits of a health intervention are referred to as **outcomes**. Health outcomes can assume any form, but the most common health outcomes are big picture items, such as hospitalizations prevented, illnesses avoided, or deaths averted (as opposed to little picture items, such as stomachaches reduced).

The first question that should pop into mind when speaking of the cost-effectiveness of a particular intervention such as mammography aimed at improving a health outcome is, Relative to what? Mammography will certainly appear cost-effective if we compare it to a total body scan for breast cancer. But it might not be cost-effective relative to educating women to perform breast self-examination in the shower on a regular basis. The intervention to which you are comparing the intervention of interest is called the **competing alternative**.

The Competing Alternative

Improvements in health states and improvements in length of life do not always go hand-in-hand. For instance, we perform mammography even though the procedure produces discomfort. Likewise, we provide steroids to patients with asthma even though this medication can be harmful over the long term. Such complications shouldn't be a deterrent. The whole point of cost-effectiveness, after all, is to examine the optimal course of action when there is considerable uncertainty. (Otherwise why bother with the analysis in the first place?)

Uncertainty also arises when one intervention is slightly more effective but costs considerably more than the competing alternative. In these instances, one cannot know whether more lives will be saved by spending the money on the more effective intervention or by purchasing the cheaper, less effective alternative and then spending the money saved on another lifesaving modality.

Virtually all health interventions cost something up front. But they also affect the amount of money spent on future medical care. For instance, a woman who is found to have breast cancer at an early stage will likely incur the cost of hospitalization and surgery in addition to the mammography, but the cancer may be cured, averting the future cost of more severe disease. Thus, mammography can produce value by averting disease and future costs. In short, the overall cost and overall effectiveness of any given alternative strategy are not often apparent on first glance.

So what is the net (overall) cost of mammography, and how much benefit can we expect? To answer this question, we first want a sense of how much of an improvement in health states we'll get from mammography over the long term.

Health States

While health outcomes such as deaths are concrete overarching measures of health, it is also important to examine more specific improvements in one's state of health, such as reduced pain or improved ability to walk. Specific states of health are quite logically referred to as **health states**. (Whoever said cost-effectiveness was difficult?)

Figure 1.1 shows how a health intervention improves health states. Here, we see that people having an asthma attack arrive at the emergency room with difficulty breathing (health state 1). The health intervention is to provide intravenous steroids and aerosolized medications to help such patients breathe. Typically, patients experience dramatic improvements in breathing once treated (health state 2).

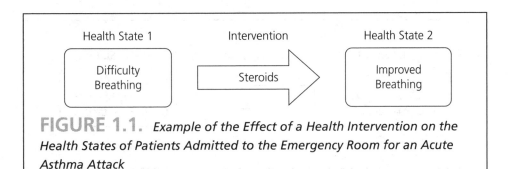

FIGURE 1.1. *Example of the Effect of a Health Intervention on the Health States of Patients Admitted to the Emergency Room for an Acute Asthma Attack*

Simple. So why the fuss? We wish to first think about this in very simplistic terms because we will later need to think about the various ways in which health states change when a medical intervention occurs, which can be somewhat complex. Collectively, improvements in health states add up to improvements in one's **health status**.

Health Status

A person's health status is the sum of his or her health states. If someone can jog and isn't anxious or depressed, we might say that the person has an excellent health status based on those two health states alone.

In a cost-effectiveness analysis, a researcher gathers information on the ways in which a health intervention changes the average health status of a group of people alongside costs (Figure 1.2). Imagine for a moment you are evaluating a treatment for bacterial pneumonia and comparing it to no treatment at all. In Figure 1.2, "health status 1" represents the collective health states of untreated people, and "health status 2" represents the collective health states of treated people.

Suppose were looking at treatment of bacterial pneumonia with antibiotics. Someone with bacterial pneumonia might have pain with breathing and a fever and be confined to bed. Someone who has been treated would have less pain and less fever and might be able to get around. In other words, the treated person would experience an improvement in health status.

Because health status is an amorphous concept, there is no direct way to measure it. Instead, cost-effectiveness analysis examines the quantity of life alongside a measure of the quality of life associated with a given health status. The point of a cost-effectiveness analysis is therefore to estimate what an improvement in health status will produce in terms of quality and quantity of life and how much it will cost to achieve these improvements.

We must also look at how health status (the collection of health states) changes over time. For instance, suppose you are again at your job at a major cancer society, and you are trying to decide whether to recommend screening mammography. Cancer evolves over many years. So we'll want to know how it will affect everything from a patient's ability to perform daily activities to her mental health as time goes on.

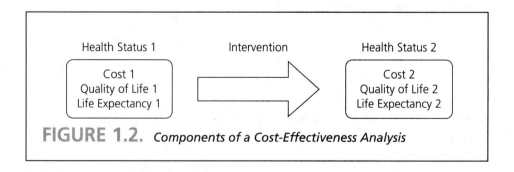

FIGURE 1.2. *Components of a Cost-Effectiveness Analysis*

Take another look at Figure 1.2 The quality of life in health status 1 for women screened for breast cancer is higher over the short term than it is in health status 2. Women in health status 1 have not undergone the pain of having their breast squeezed between two metal plates and do not have to face the pain and suffering associated with the diagnosis (or a misdiagnosis) of breast cancer if it is detected. In fact, since the cancer is producing no symptoms and the women do not know that they have breast cancer, they will be as subjectively healthy as anyone else over the short term. But the women in health state 2 (undetected cancer) may not have to face the pain and suffering associated with advanced breast cancer in the future.

Finally, the length of life is shorter for women who have not received a mammogram (life expectancy 1) than those who have (life expectancy 2). This is a critical factor that must be considered in any cost-effectiveness analysis. But what do we do with all this information on health status and life expectancy? Enter the **quality-adjusted life year (QALY)**.

The Quality-Adjusted Life Year

Consider the nuanced changes in the quality of life that occur when a person with diabetes is given a medication to lower blood sugar. At first, the patient has to take a pill and may think of herself as sicker than she did before being given the prescription. But over time, this pill might prevent a myocardial infarction, which would have a grave impact on the person's perception of her health and her ability to get around or to do other things she enjoys. In other words, it affects many different dimensions of this person's health, or many different health states. Together, real-world improvements in these health states, along with their effect on life expectancy that occur when a health intervention is applied, constitute the effectiveness of that intervention.

Just to drill the point home, a health outcome (such as a myocardial infarction) leads to changes in one's health states (ability to walk, work, or even to have sex), which in turn affect the person's quantity and quality of life. If we could somehow combine a measure of quality of life with a measure of quantity of life, we would be just about set in terms of measuring the effectiveness of any given health intervention.

As it turns out, we have just such a thing: the quality-adjusted life year, more affectionately known as a QALY, is a year of life lived in perfect health. At any given age, the average number of years we can expect to live is our life expectancy. Therefore, the average number of QALYs we can expect to live is our **quality-adjusted life expectancy (QALE)**. QALE is the average number of years one can expect to live in a state of perfect health. Throughout this book, you'll become increasingly familiar with what a QALY is, how it is calculated, and how it is used. For now, just accept that it is a year of perfect health.

Costs

For a moment, let's consider the changes in costs associated with mammography. The total cost of mammography includes those costs associated with the mammogram as well as future medical costs incurred as a result of this screening test. These future costs will include the value of lost work and the medical costs associated with treating cancer that was detected early.

Failing to provide a screening test also costs something. These costs include those associated with treating breast cancer that is so advanced that it is self-evident to the patient or is easily detectable on physical examination. People with advanced breast cancer will incur higher medical costs and miss more work than will those who were diagnosed early in the course of illness. All of these costs must ultimately be considered.

When comparing mammography to no mammography, the difference in costs, morbidity, and mortality is captured in the *incremental cost-effectiveness ratio*. This tells you how much you will need to spend to realize a unit gain in effectiveness.

THE COST-EFFECTIVENESS RATIO

Ratios put medical information into perspective. For instance, if a physician knows that there are 180,000 new cases of breast cancer a year in the United States, she will not be able to provide much information to a woman worried about developing that disease. If the physician knows that there are 11 new cases per 10,000 women each year, she will have a much better idea of how to communicate the risk.

Similarly, the cost-effectiveness ratio provides the consumers of our research with information that more readily allows comparisons. In fact, it provides a ton of information in one single number. The cost-effectiveness ratio not only provides information on cost, improvements in health status, and changes in life expectancy, but it also has a built-in comparison: it tells you how much you will spend to buy additional health relative to the competing alternative.

Let's take an example. Suppose you are working for a pharmaceutical company that just came out with a powerful new antibiotic for treating staphylococcus infection, Staphbegone. It is more effective than other antibiotics at saving life, but it's also much more expensive than what is now being used, Staphbeilln. But it will also get people out of the hospital faster, so it will reduce hospitalization costs and produce improvements in health-related quality of life.

We want to compare Staphbegone to Staphbeilln. We put Staphbeilln on the right-hand side of the equation because it is less effective. (This ensures that the ratio will be positive if the intervention costs money but improves health and negative if the intervention saves money and improves health.) If we call the old drug "intervention 1" and the new drug "intervention 2," the incremental cost-effectiveness ratio takes the form:

$$\frac{(\text{Cost of intervention 2 } - \text{ Cost of intervention 1})}{(\text{Quality-adjusted life expectancy 2 } - \text{ Quality-adjusted life expectancy 1})} \quad (1.1)$$

Here, quality-adjusted life expectancy is used in the denominator because this is the standard unit of effectiveness (more on standardization in the next chapter). However, in some cases (also discussed in the next chapter), other measures of effectiveness might be used. Some economists call these additional costs and effectiveness values

marginal values. In cost-effectiveness speak, they are generally referred to as **incremental values**.

Now, you should have a general idea of what cost-effectiveness is. You should also have an idea of what the incremental cost-effectiveness ratio means. In the next section, we move from what cost-effectiveness is to why cost-effectiveness analysis is a critical part of any well-functioning society.

EXERCISES 1 AND 2

1. Suppose that a complete course of Staphbegone costs $12,000 and a complete course of Staphbeilln costs $4,000. The average hospitalization costs $1,000 per day. Patients given Staphbegone have an average length of hospitalization of 5 days and Staphbeilln have an average hospitalization of 10 days. What is the incremental cost of Staphbegone?

2. Persons given Staphbegone have a higher survival rate than those given Staphbeilln. On average, those given Staphbegone can expect to go on to have a quality-adjusted life expectancy of 35 QALYs, while those given Staphbeilln go on to live 34.5 QALYs. Using the answer from exercise 1.2, what is the incremental cost-effectiveness of Staphbegone?

TIPS AND TRICKS

Answers to all self-study questions are presented in Appendix A.

WHY CONDUCT COST-EFFECTIVENESS ANALYSIS?

There are a number of ways to prevent or treat most diseases. For instance, breast cancer can be detected by self-examination, examination by a medical practitioner, screening mammography, ultrasound, spiral CT, or MRI. It is also possible to compare different levels of intensity of a single health intervention. For example, screening mammography might be performed every six months, every year, or every two years. Each of these competing alternatives is associated with a different effectiveness and a different cost. In the real world, many different approaches are used to diagnose or treat disease (Wennberg and Gittelsohn, 1982), some by crackpot medical practitioners.

Many students of cost-effectiveness analysis rightly question the logic of choosing interventions based on both cost and effectiveness criteria rather than effectiveness alone. After all, it is often argued, shouldn't we purchase the best treatments regardless of their costs? In the first section of this chapter, we saw that there is an almost infinite number of life-saving expenditures, including some combination of screening modalities. The question, then, is, Which ones can we afford? To answer this question, let's first consider what we mean by *cost* and what we mean by *effectiveness*.

Costs Matter

Even when the most effective modality is known, it may have unforeseen effects on human life if its use takes vital resources from other social programs. First, consider your personal budget. Suppose that you make $2,000 a month. Now suppose that your rent, minimum food purchases, basic utilities, and transportation come to $1,800. You could spend some of the $200 on going out to the movies and save the rest. Alternatively, you could live it up and go out to a fancy dinner and the theater five nights a month and live without electricity; go on an expensive vacation and not pay your rent; or blow the whole wad on that haute couture suit you've always wanted. Some of us can accept that it's not possible to consume everything we want. But when the goods and services we are consuming define who lives and who dies, the choices become much more difficult.

Consider the case of a tiny country with 100 people and a total health budget of $10,000 per year. If the country paid for expensive organ transplants, it could spend its entire budget on one person, leaving nothing for clean water, vaccinations, primary care, or other medical services that greatly prolong the quality and quantity of life for everyone in the country. If it instead spent $1,000 per year to keep vaccinations up to date, $7,000 per year for all needed antibiotics and basic primary care, and $2,000 per year on emergency surgery, many more lives would be saved. The value of goods and services in their best alternative use is the **opportunity cost** of an investment, such as a medical intervention.

Thus, just as your electricity bill has an opportunity cost, so too does vaccination.

FOR EXAMPLE

The Case for Education as a Health Expenditure

Basic schooling is thought to greatly reduce morbidity and mortality in both the industrialized and developing context. Education provides the cognitive skills and the social credentials needed for survival and adaptation to any ecological niche (Wilkinson, 1999). For instance, middle-class neighborhoods tend to have lower rates of crime victimization, access to healthier foods, and better housing. None of this is likely without an adequate education. Similarly, cognitive skills allow people to better assess hazards (such as taking the train instead of a bus in India), and may even reduce errors in medication dosage or compliance with medical prescriptions. As it turns out, education not only saves lives; it saves money (Muennig and Woolf, 2007). Therefore, it can be argued that basic education should be prioritized over the provision of basic medical services when resources are slim (Muennig and Woolf, 2007).

In circumstances where health funds are budgeted (and therefore fixed), cost-effectiveness analysis can provide information on how to realize the largest health gains with the money that you have (Gold, Siegel, Russell, and Weinstein, 1996; Ubel, DeKay, Baron, and Asch 1996). For instance, in a country with a national health system, interventions can be ranked in order of their cost-effectiveness. If we know how much will be spent on each health intervention in total, it becomes possible to go down the list until the money runs out. This is also known as **appropriate technology utilization**; if a government barely has money to pay for vaccination (an appropriate technology), it does not make sense to pay for heart-lung transplants (a technology that is inappropriate given the budgetary constraints).

The use of appropriate technology isn't always popular. A person who needs a heart and lung transplant and is dying in the hospital evokes more sympathy than the unseen hundreds of people who might benefit from all of the vaccines that could be purchased with the same sum of cash. However, in the absence of sufficient funding to cover all known treatments for all known diseases, prioritizing expensive and less effective interventions will ultimately lead to more illness and death.

In the United States, medical care is almost never denied to anyone who can afford it, and there is no absolute cap on how much is spent on health care. In this setting, cost-effectiveness analysis provides clinicians, policymakers, and insurers with general guidelines on which interventions might generally be preferable. For instance, an intervention that costs $100,000 for each QALY it produces relative to the next most effective alternative might be seen as expensive by some, but might be purchased by others.

While highly anecdotal, this lack of an emphasis on cost-effectiveness likely provides a partial explanation for why the United States spends around twice as much on health care as the next biggest spender but ranks twenty-fifth among developing nations in terms of life expectancy (World Health Organization, 2006).

In developing nations, where government health budgets may be as low as five dollars per person, the need for cost-effectiveness analysis becomes critical (Attaran and Sachs, 2001). When budgets are small, the use of inappropriate technologies can greatly increase mortality in the population as a whole. Why more so than in industrialized nations? Simply because forgoing the least expensive and most effective interventions such as vaccinations produces more harm than forgoing interventions that produce less spectacular gains and cost more, such as dialysis. The basis for such decisions therefore has at least as much to do with its effectiveness at a population level as its cost.

Effectiveness Versus Efficacy

Usually tests, treatments, or interventions are measured in terms of their **efficacy**. Efficacy reveals how a test, treatment, or intervention works under experimental conditions. Experiments tend to work better under the watchful eye of researchers in a controlled laboratory setting than in the real world. Subjects are watched to make sure they take their medications and that laboratory specimens are properly frozen and shipped immediately for testing. In the real world, conditions tend to be less exacting.

Experiments that measure efficacy also tend to look at only short-term outcomes. There is usually one test that is known to detect the most cases, a treatment that has the highest cure rate, or public health interventions that are most likely to prevent a disease. Each of these is often thought of as the most efficacious option for preventing or treating disease. But can we say that the use of the most efficacious interventions will detect the most cases of disease, have the highest rate of treatment success, or prevent the most diseases in the real world?

Often the answer is no. Not only are tests performed differently or medications taken in different doses in the real world, but a number of other things happen as well. For instance, screening tests and treatments are sometimes associated with hidden dangers. As we saw in the screening mammography example, a false-positive mammogram can lead to unnecessary surgery and psychological stress.

Moreover, most treatments can produce debilitating or fatal side effects in a fraction of the people taking them. Therefore, when we examine the effectiveness of a treatment at extending human life expectancy, we have to consider that the treatment can prolong life in one way but reduce life expectancy in another way. Thus, the real-world effects may be smaller than the efficacy of the treatment would suggest. **Effectiveness** indicates how well such tests, treatments, or programs perform in the real world.

By providing data on effectiveness, cost-effectiveness analysis provides information on how interventions are likely to work in everyday use. While supplementing cereal grains with the vitamin folate may greatly reduce neural tube defects in newborns, it may also lead to the underdiagnosis of vitamin B_{12} deficiency among poor or elderly populations (Haddix, Teutsch, Shaffer, and Dunet, 1996). When vitamin B_{12} deficiency is not diagnosed and treated early, it too can lead to severe neurological complications. Thus, the efficacy of a given treatment in preventing a disease may not be representative of its overall effectiveness at preventing death due to that disease.

THE REFERENCE CASE ANALYSIS

Cost-effectiveness analyses can take many subtly different forms. Consider the case of a local health department that wishes to know the cost of screening people for tuberculosis in its clinics. It may examine the cost per case of active tuberculosis prevented when patients are screened in its clinics (relative to not providing these screening exams). This type of analysis would furnish the health department with information useful for making specific internal decisions, such as whether it is worthwhile to spend money on such programs. However, it would not provide a good deal of information on the overall benefits of screening to the population it serves because it does not provide any information on the ill effects of tuberculosis itself.

Or the health department may wish to expand the analysis in order to obtain information on both the cost-effectiveness of its operations and its broader mission of improving the longevity of the population it serves. For instance, it may wish to determine the cost of the program per year of life saved as well as the cost per case prevented. This would also provide information for internal decision making and on how the programs are benefiting the populations that they serve.

Finally, tuberculosis is a severe disease that can require burdensome treatments and long stints in hospitals (sometimes in an isolated room), and it can have an impact on people's quality of life. The health department may therefore also wish to examine the cost of tuberculosis screening relative to improvements in the quality and quantity of life of the population it serves. This type of information would allow them to assess the impact of tuberculosis on mortality. It would also allow them to compare the cost of tuberculosis screening programs to programs that predominantly affect the quality of life, such as mental health programs.

While some health events, such as high-rise construction accidents, predominantly affect the quantity of life, others, such as repetitive stress injuries at work, predominantly affect the quality of life. When a measure of quality of life is added to a cost-effectiveness analysis, it becomes possible to compare health interventions across the spectrum of disease. (Recall that one QALY is a year of life lived in perfect health.)

The ability to make comparisons across different diseases opens up the possibility of standardizing cost-effectiveness analyses, so that the incremental gains associated with virtually any intervention can be compared with those of another. If the health department conducted its analysis based on the cost per active case of tuberculosis prevented, it would provide some information on how the new intervention compares with what it is doing now. But it wouldn't be able to compare its new intervention with other programs in the health department because the denominator is different. If it used life expectancy, the denominator would be the same. Therefore, it could compare the cost per life saved of the tuberculosis program with a program that aimed to prevent window falls.

But you would still miss the boat. A program designed to reduce repetitive stress injuries at work wouldn't save many lives. Therefore, no matter how good the program is, it will always seem less cost-effective than a program designed to prevent window falls. Here again, the QALY saves the day. By comparing interventions across a term that captures both quality and quantity of life, it becomes possible to measure the relative cost-effectiveness of each program in the health department—provided that costs, quality measures, and life years gained are all calculated in a similar way in each of the analyses. Under these conditions, it is possible to compare the incremental cost per QALY gained for health interventions as different as vaccination and migraine prevention. Of course, you need a standard set of methods to refer to if you are going to do this. This more or less standardized set of methods is called the **reference case analysis** (Gold, Siegel, Russell, and Weinstein, 1996).

The use of disparate approaches to cost-effectiveness analysis sometimes leads to widely different study results. For example, in the introduction to their book, the Panel on Cost-Effectiveness in Health and Medicine notes that the published cost-effectiveness of screening mammography for the detection of breast cancer varies from cost savings to $80,000 per life saved (Gold, Siegel, Russell, and Weinstein, 1996). The panel set methodological standards for conducting cost-effectiveness analyses in hopes of closing that gap. And the reference case was born.

The reference case is the most comprehensive type of cost-effectiveness analysis. It requires the use of QALYs as the unit of effectiveness to ensure that all studies have comparable outcomes. The reference case also requires that the study include all costs (regardless of who pays) that are likely to be relevant. In this book we focus on reference case analyses because it is important to know the rules of the reference case and because it provides the most comprehensive tool kit for conducting any type of cost-effectiveness analysis you wish.

FOR EXAMPLE

What's in a Name?

A lot of fuss is made over the distinction between *health* interventions and *medical* interventions (Gold, Siegel, Russell, and Weinstein, 1996). *Health* generally refers to public health programs, such as the provision of clean water or laws requiring grains to be fortified with vitamins. *Medical interventions* specifically refer to things that medical providers do, such as selecting the most appropriate antibiotic. In practice, the distinction is blurry. For instance, checking blood pressure might be considered a health intervention if it is done as part of a screening program, but a medical intervention if it is done to ensure that a patient is receiving the proper dosage of medication. In this book, we usually refer to both types of interventions under the general heading of "health."

Why would you want to conduct any type of cost-effectiveness analysis besides the reference case analysis? Consider the health department used as an example at the beginning of this section. If the department is interested only in internal decision making, a reference case analysis would provide superfluous information, such as private sector costs and patient costs. Therefore, a reference case analysis is not necessarily the best approach in all situations. (For more information, see "A Note on Methods" in the Preface to this book.)

You now should have a sense of what cost-effectiveness is, why it is important, and who it is important for. In the next section, we move on to how cost-effectiveness analysis is used to make policy decisions in health.

COST-EFFECTIVENESS ANALYSIS AND POLICY

We have noted that cost-effectiveness analyses are primarily used to compare different strategies for preventing or treating a single disease (such as tuberculosis). In addition, they can be used to maximize the quality and quantity of life within a given budget. In this section, we briefly explore how policy decisions are sometimes made using cost-effectiveness analyses, as well as some of the controversies that have arisen as a result of such policy decisions.

Prioritizing Health Interventions

It is possible to use cost-effectiveness analysis to purchase the most health under a fixed budget. If the incremental cost-effectiveness of everything that is done in medicine were known, we would have a sense of the opportunity cost of any health investment we might make (Jamison, Mosley, Measham, and Bobadilla, 1993. It would therefore be possible to list all interventions in a table and then draw a line between what is and is not affordable. When incremental cost-effectiveness ratios for different interventions are listed in a table, it is sometimes called a **league table** (Mauskopf, Rutten, and Schonfeld, 2003).

FOR EXAMPLE

Cost-Effectiveness in Developing Countries

Nowhere else is cost-effectiveness analysis more important than in developing countries. With annual health budgets as low as five dollars per person, efficiency is critical. Recognizing the need for better health purchases, the World Health Organization developed CHOosing Interventions that are Cost-Effective (CHOICE). CHOICE is a program that contains information on costs, mortality, quality-of-life measures, and completed cost-effectiveness analyses for each region of the world (http://www.who.int/choice/en/).

League tables can also be used to place a given intervention in context. For instance, suppose we know that mammography costs $30,000 per QALY gained relative to no mammography. We can't be sure whether this is expensive or cheap relative to other things done in medicine. However, suppose we know that treating an otherwise fatal bacterial pneumonia with a commonly used antibiotic costs $25,000 per QALY gained relative to no treatment. Then we know that $30,000 per QALY gained for mammography is in the ballpark of a treatment that most would agree should not be denied. But if treating bacterial pneumonia were found to cost $300 per QALY gained and heart-lung transplants in active chain smokers were found to cost $15,000 per QALY, then perhaps mammography wouldn't be such a reasonable thing to do.

Let's take a look at how else a league table might be used. Table 1.1 represents a hypothetical league table for a village in Malawi with a total health budget of $58,000. In this table, we rank a number of interventions by their incremental cost-effectiveness ratio relative to not providing the treatment at all. This ratio tells how much it costs to buy one year of perfect health.

TABLE 1.1. **Hypothetical League Table for a Village in Malawi with a $58,000 Health Budget**

Intervention	Incremental Cost-Effectiveness Ratio[A]	Size of Affected Population	Total Cost per Year
Measles vaccine	$375	5,000	$15,000
Sexually transmitted disease treatment	$420	300	$2,100
Pneumonia treatment	$428	150	$1,800
Mosquito nets	$846	22,000	$44,000
HIV treatment	$3,000	100	$30,000
Totals			$92,900

[A]The reference intervention is to do nothing.

If we know the size of the affected population and the total cost of the intervention, we know how much we will spend per year on any given strategy and the total number of QALYs we'll save. In this case, we only have $58,000, so we can't even provide the first four treatments, which collectively cost nearly $63,000. We might use this table to advocate for more funding or to figure out how we might reassess our interventions. For instance, prioritizing bed nets for children, who have not yet developed immunity to malaria, may be more cost-effective than providing them to family members who are older and less likely to succumb to the disease.

EXERCISES 3 AND 4

3. How many QALYs will $1,000 worth of measles vaccine purchase in this village?

4. A nongovernmental organization geared toward providing mosquito nets comes to a similar village in Malawi to the one represented in Table 1.1. This village has no health budget but wishes to provide $1,000 worth of mosquito nets. How many QALYs will be forgone as a result of spending the money on nets rather than on the measles vaccine?

However tempting it might be to create a list of interventions based on their cost-effectiveness, decisions surrounding the allocation of social resources cannot be made based on numbers alone. For example, HIV medications in Table 1.1 purchase a large amount of health for a small group of people, which might not be seen as fair for the village as a whole. Cost-effectiveness analysis does not provide ethical information; it is just one handy tool policymakers might use when deciding on which interventions they will fund (Gold, Siegel, Russell, and Weinstein, 1996). (Other examples of league tables can be found at: http://www.tufts-nemc.org/cearegistry/. For further discussion, including the limitations of league tables, please see Mauskopf (2003).

FOR EXAMPLE

Chile's Story: How to Succeed by Not Being Cost-Effective

Chile is attempting to create a national health plan, called "Plan Auge," that partly uses a league table to achieve its policy objectives. The idea is to start covering a small number of conditions and then scale up the program as time goes on. Rather than choose the most cost-effective interventions to start with, however, those who designed the plan deliberately chose inefficient but heart-warming treatments, such as chemotherapy for children. The result? An astounding success: the president invited the cured children and other patients for a press conference to tout the success of the program. This single media event defeated the resistance of insurance companies and the national medical association. At the time of printing this book, the list was up to over fifty conditions (A. Infante, personal communication, 2006).

Do Cost-Effectiveness Analyses Actually Change the Way Things Are Done?

Examples of policy decisions that have been influenced by cost-effectiveness analysis include strategies for reducing parasitic infections in immigrant populations (Muennig, Pallin, Sell, and Chan, 1999), conducting cervical cancer screening among low-income elderly women (Fahs, Mandelblatt, Schechter, and Muller, 1992), and adding folate to cereal grains in the United States (Haddix, Teutsch, Shaffer, and Dunet, 1996). These studies appear to have sparked changes in the way that patients received medical care in local health departments, changes in Medicare reimbursement policies, and changes in the rules set by the U.S. Department of Agriculture. Still, although Canada, Australia, and a number of European countries use cost-effectiveness to help decide what should be paid for and what should not, Medicare has not yet officially incorporated cost-effectiveness analysis into its payment policies (Neumann, Rosen, and Weinstein, 2005).

Cost-effectiveness analyses can also lead to policy changes with broader implications than the authors intended. For instance, when supplementing cereal grains was found to be a cost-effective strategy for preventing neural tube defects in the United States, cost-effectiveness analysis not only helped convince the food industry that it was worth the cost, but other countries also considered similar interventions (Schaller and Olson, 1996; Wynn and Wynn, 1998).

Cost-effectiveness analysis has also proven to be a controversial tool when used without taking the broader social implications of health interventions into account. For example, in the state of Oregon in the United States, cost-effectiveness analysis was used to prioritize health interventions paid for by the state government using a league table. Those interventions deemed unaffordable were not paid for, creating a large statewide and national outcry from groups denied treatment on these grounds (Oregon Health Services Commission, 1991; Oregon Office for Health Policy and Research, 2001).

These real-world examples highlight some of the promises and pitfalls of cost-effectiveness analysis for policy. Students embarking on this endeavor may one day find themselves facing tough ethical decisions for which there is no right answer. For instance, you may be working for a government that wishes to base immigration policies on preexisting conditions for applicants. Or you might be working for an insurance company that wishes to deny an effective treatment based on its cost-effectiveness. In such instances, consultation with an ethicist is paramount.

CHAPTER

2

PRINCIPLES OF COST-EFFECTIVENESS ANALYSIS

OVERVIEW

SO FAR, you have learned what cost-effectiveness is and how it is used to make policy. This chapter introduces the basic concepts behind cost-effectiveness analysis. We explore the different types of analyses, how costs are tabulated, how health-related quality of life is measured, and how QALYs are generated. You will also learn how to interpret cost-effectiveness ratios in more detail.

THE PERSPECTIVE OF A COST-EFFECTIVENESS ANALYSIS

Terry Jones, the chief executive officer of a large insurance company, has received hundreds of requests for contraceptive reimbursement from the company's enrollees. He is interested in improving the company's services for the enrollees but is concerned that the costs might be prohibitive. Nevertheless, because the company must pay for pregnancies when they occur, reimbursing patients for contraceptives might reduce the company's expenditures on hospitalization costs.

Jones realizes that if the company does not reimburse for the birth-control pill, most of the company's clients who wish to protect themselves from pregnancy will purchase the contraceptives on their own. However, some people will have unwanted pregnancies because it was either too inconvenient or too expensive for them to purchase contraceptives. Because pregnancy occasionally results in medical complications or even death, the company's failure to pay for contraceptives could theoretically result in litigation as well. Therefore, Jones commissions an analysis examining the cost of providing contraceptives per pregnancy prevented when the insurance company pays for contraception versus a no-pay policy.

Jo Jo Thompson is the commissioner of a local health department in Saratoga, Illinois. Thompson receives a report indicating that the maternal mortality rate among low-income women in Saratoga has increased over the past year. He decides to conduct an analysis to examine whether providing contraceptives to low-income women who cannot otherwise afford them is cost-effective. Thompson wishes to know whether his health department can afford the program and whether it will be effective at reducing maternal mortality.

Finally, Tina Johanas is a U.S. senator interested in enacting legislation mandating that all insurance companies pay for contraceptives. Johanas's primary interest is to improve the quality of life of her constituents, but she is also concerned about the overall impact of the proposed legislation on the health care system. Therefore, she commissions a cost-effectiveness analysis examining the incremental cost per QALY gained when insurance companies pay for contraception relative to the cost per QALY gained of the current policy of letting insurance companies decide whether to pay for contraceptives.

In the analysis conducted from the perspective of the insurance company headed by Jones, the relevant question is whether the company pays for all of the contraceptives or none of the contraceptives. Jones decides not to include any costs incurred by patients in the analysis because such costs do not appear on his company's budget. He would be interested in knowing whether paying for contraceptives might reduce pregnancy-associated costs, because such costs account for a portion of his company's expenditures.

Commissioner Thompson is interested in costs specific to the health department. He wishes to include only medical services and goods for which the health department will pay. These might include the cost of medical services that occur in health department clinics and the cost of the contraceptive itself. Unlike Jones, Commissioner Thompson does not wish to include the costs associated with pregnancies that occur among privately insured women since they do not appear on his balance sheet.

Finally, Senator Johanas is worried about the overall costs of her legislation to everyone in society. She wishes to ensure that the interests of health departments, insurance companies, and regular citizens are met. Therefore, she wishes to include all costs relevant to enacting the legislation or failing to enact the legislation. Moreover,

Johanas is worried about the overall health and well-being of her constituents rather than just the number of pregnancies prevented. Because unwanted pregnancy can cause emotional as well as physical harm, she wishes to ensure that the overall quality of life of women with unwanted pregnancies is accounted for in the analysis.

The party interested in the study can have an influence on which costs and which effectiveness outcomes are included in an analysis. When a particular organization includes only costs and outcomes relevant to its needs, the analysis is said to have been conducted from that party's perspective. For example, when the study applies only to a government agency, the study is said to assume a **governmental perspective**. When the study applies to society as a whole, it is said to assume a **societal perspective**. Table 2.1 illustrates the different types of costs that might be included in a study from the perspective of an insurance company, a government agency, or society as a whole.

In Table 2.1, each of these three entities is paying for the cost of the contraceptive, medical visits, and hospitalization. Because insurance companies do not have to compensate patients for their time or pay transportation costs or environmental costs, these costs would not be included in a study that assumes the perspective of the insurance company. However, the government would be interested in some of these costs. For example, because the local government disproportionately hires low-income women, some of the women seeking contraception might be government employees and will take time off from work to receive medical care.

TABLE 2.1. **Costs Included in a Cost-Effectiveness Analysis of Free Contraception, Conducted from Three Perspectives**

Cost	Insurance	Government	Society
Contraceptive pill	All costs	All costs	All costs
Medical visit	All costs	All costs	All costs
Hospitalization	All costs	All costs	All costs
Patient time	No costs	Some costs	All costs
Transportation	No costs	Some costs	All costs
Environment	No costs	All costs	All costs
Education system	No costs	Most costs	All costs

From the societal perspective, all costs must be included regardless of who pays for them. "Society" refers to everyone who might be affected by the intervention. Thus, costs relevant to the government, employers, patients, insurance companies, and anyone or anything else should be included as long as they are likely to be large enough to make a difference in the analysis. Usually the term *society* refers to everything within the borders of a country (Drummond, O'Brien, Stoddart, and Torrance, 2005).

The societal perspective, the most important, can be a bit confusing. For instance, suppose that we are looking at the cost-effectiveness of shifting the responsibility for paying for vaccines from the private sector to the government from the societal perspective. Suppose further that we anticipate that 30 million children will receive the vaccine in any given year. If it costs, all things included, $15 to vaccinate a child and 30 million children are vaccinated, what is the difference in cost when the government takes over? The answer: No change in costs; we are merely shifting the $45 million in costs from private insurers to the government. If under the new program, however, there are differences in the wages of those giving the vaccines, transportation costs, and so forth, the change could be associated with higher or lower costs per vaccination.

Since different perspectives require including or excluding different costs, the only way to standardize cost-effectiveness analyses is to require that all of these analyses assume the same perspective. For this reason, among others, the reference case scenario of the Panel on Cost-Effectiveness in Health and Medicine requires that the societal perspective be adopted (Gold, Siegel, Russell, and Weinstein, 1996).

To publish cost-effectiveness analyses, you will generally need to include a reference case analysis so that your results can be placed in the context of other studies. When all costs are included, it is a simple task to exclude some of the costs not of interest to one party or another. This way, you can easily add another perspective (for example, governmental as well as societal) to your study.

In the insurance company's case, it might conduct a reference case analysis and then calculate cost-effectiveness ratios from the company's perspective by leaving out the costs mentioned in Table 2.1 that aren't relevant. If the company were to publish the study in the medical literature (perhaps to attract attention to its good deeds), it could simply present the reference case results along with the results of interest to the company.

CAPTURING COSTS

Before we go on, take another look at equation 1.1 from Chapter One:

$$\frac{(\text{Cost of intervention 2} - \text{Cost of intervention 1})}{(\text{Quality-adjusted life expectancy 2} - \text{Quality-adjusted life expectancy 1})} \quad (2.1)$$

Let's call doing nothing "intervention 1" and mammography for women over the age of 50 "intervention 2." (Remember that the more effective intervention goes on the left of the equation.) In this instance, our research question is, "What happens when women who would not otherwise have received a mammogram are given one?"

We saw in Figure 1.2 that the new intervention (in this case, mammography) moves women with breast cancer from health status 1 (undetected cancer) to health status 2 (cancer detected early). Since this is the "capturing costs" section of the book, our job here is to think only about costs. We need to consider three factors: (1) the cost associated with health state 1, (2) the costs associated with the intervention, and (3) the costs associated with health state 2.

The total cost of doing nothing is equal to the total cost of health state 1. In health state 1, women who do not have breast cancer will go on with their lives without incurring any costs whatsoever. Those who do have cancer but don't know it will incur the future costs associated with more advanced disease.

The total cost of the mammography intervention is the cost of mammography itself plus the total cost of health state 2. The total cost of health state 2 may be something less than the total cost of health state 2 because it is generally less expensive to treat less advanced disease than it is to treat more advanced disease.

The cost of medical visits, hospitalizations, X-rays, and other goods and services are referred to as **direct costs**. Consider the cost of time lost in going to the doctor's office or time spent away from the beach due to breast cancer. The Americans have the saying, "time is money," and in cost-effectiveness analysis, we attempt to place a monetary value on this time. Lost time is an **indirect cost**. Such costs are called "indirect" because they don't involve the consumption of goods or services.

While indirect costs still involve the consumption of something that is measurable (for example, the time spent doing something), there are costs that can't be easily accounted for. Such costs, referred to as **intangible costs**, are those that cannot be measured by any conventional metric. Examples of intangible costs are pain, suffering, or the monetary value of a year of healthy life. In cost-effectiveness analysis, intangible costs related to pain and suffering (quality of life) are also often referred to as **morbidity costs**, and costs related to death are sometimes called **mortality costs**.

In cost-effectiveness analysis, intangible costs are not monetized. Rather, such costs are captured in the quality-of-life measure used to calculate QALYs.

CAPTURING QUALITY

Recall that a QALY is one year of life spent in perfect health. The trick is to come up with some subjective measure of how to convert a year of life lived with disease into a year of life lived in perfect health. This is done through the use of a **health-related quality-of-life (HRQL) score**. This score is commonly referred to simply as the *HRQL score*.

The HRQL (sometimes abbreviated as HRQoL) score measures the effect of a disease on the way a person enjoys life. This includes the way illness affects a person's

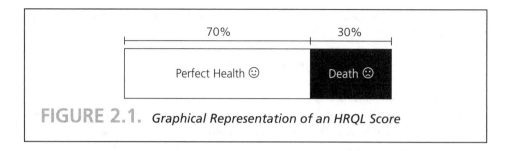

FIGURE 2.1. *Graphical Representation of an HRQL Score*

ability to live free of pain, work productively, and interact with loved ones. In other words, the HRQL score translates a person's perception of his or her quality of life with a particular illness into a number.

For example, on a scale from 0 to 1, individuals who consider themselves to be in perfect health would rate their life as a 1, and someone who would just as soon be dead might rate his or her life as a 0. Another person with a chronic debilitating disease might rate life as a 0.7, indicating that she values her life as worth only seven-tenths of a year of life lived in perfect health (see Figure 2.1).

In this example, one year of perfect health is therefore simply 0.7 × 1 year = 0.7 QALY. Two years in this state is 0.7 × 2 years = 1.4 QALYs. In other words, while the QALY represents a year of perfect health, the HRQL score represents the proportion of time lived in perfect health.

You will learn how one comes by this proportion in Chapter Seven. For now, let's leave it at this: it's probably more accurate to place a 0 to 1 value on the trade-off between life and death than it is to place a monetary value on the trade-off. Therefore, we use this number rather than a dollar value.

Aha! Now you know why the HRQL score is discussed within a section of the book about costs. Let's take a second to look at an example of how this is used. Before you do, close your eyes, clear your head, and recall just three things: (1) the HRQL score tells you what proportion of your time is spent in the equivalent of perfect health; (2) the QALY is a year of life spent in perfect health; and (3) one year at an HRQL of 0.7 is equal to 0.7 QALYs.

Suppose that we are evaluating a new drug that greatly reduces the morbidity associated with adult-onset diabetes. Suppose further that although this new drug has a dramatic effect on morbidity, it has no effect on mortality. We wish to compare this new drug with current medications. If we want to know how this new drug might change the total QALYs lived from the average age of onset for diabetes (67 years) to the average age of death (77 years) in a hypothetical group of women, we would add up the differences in QALYs lived each year (see Table 2.2).

The total number of years each group of women would have lived is the same (10 years). However, when quality of life is considered, the women without treatment would have gained just 6.2 QALYs. The treated women gained 8.6 QALYs

TABLE 2.2. **Hypothetical Differences in Health-Related Quality of Life over Ten Years for Diabetic Women and Women in Perfect Health**

Year	Diabetic Women	Treated Women
1	0.8	0.9
2	0.8	0.9
3	0.7	0.9
4	0.8	0.9
5	0.6	0.9
6	0.6	0.9
7	0.5	0.8
8	0.6	0.8
9	0.4	0.8
10	0.4	0.8
Total QALYs	6.2	8.6

over those 10 years. Therefore, although their life was just as long, the treated women experience a gain in years of perfect health equal to 8.6 QALY − 6.2 QALYs = 2.4 QALYs.

Now let's think about this on a larger scale. Appendix B contains life tables for the U.S. population, which include life expectancy at a given age. If the average HRQL at birth is 0.82 and the average life expectancy is 77.5, how many QALYs does the average American live? This is a matter of simple multiplication: $77.5 \times 0.82 = 63.6$ QALYs.

In Chapter Seven, we will see that the way an HRQL score is measured can bias the calculation of QALYs. Because there is no perfect way to measure a person's HRQL score and because the HRQL can affect the way in which denominator "costs" are counted, it is important that HRQL scores are obtained and used in a consistent way. In fact, the use of something as subjective as an HRQL score affects the overall usefulness of reference case cost-effectiveness analyses (Gold, Siegel, Russell, and Weinstein, 1996; Gold and Muennig, 2002). Still, the only way to compare different interventions across different diseases is to include HRQL in the cost-effectiveness analysis.

The HRQL score is meant to capture most or all morbidity and mortality (intangible) costs. Some indirect costs, namely, those associated with **lost productivity** and **leisure time**, are also captured in the HRQL score. Illness can affect the quality and quantity of work a person performs, as well as a person's ability to enjoy his or her work. When people undergo the mental exercises needed to obtain HRQL scores, they tend to consider the impact that the illness might have on their productivity, as well as their ability to enjoy life outside work. Because of this, if we added an estimate of the patient's lost productivity and leisure time, we would be double-counting (once in the numerator and once in the denominator of the cost-effectiveness ratio).

While the time spent recovering from an illness is theoretically captured in the HRQL score, the time spent receiving treatment is not (Gold, Siegel, Russell, and Weinstein, 1996). Costs associated with receiving treatment must be included in the numerator of the cost-effectiveness ratio. Although visits to the doctor do not cause (that much) pain and suffering, recovering from an illness does, so the former goes in the numerator and the latter in the denominator. The time costs of caregivers, coworkers, or others who are not afflicted with the disease (and thus do not physically suffer) are also captured as costs in the numerator.

TIPS AND TRICKS

As a general rule, if a cost is associated with pain and suffering, it is included in the denominator of the cost-effectiveness ratio. If it is not associated with pain and suffering, it is included in the numerator of the cost-effectiveness ratio.

The use of QALYs allows researchers to combine the effects of quantity of life (for example, years of life gained by an intervention) with quality of life in a single measure. But how is something as subjective as quality measured, and how are measures of quantity and quality of life combined? In Chapter Seven, we will learn how quality is measured in cost-effectiveness analysis, and we will then learn how QALYs are calculated in Chapter Eight.

Exhibit 2.1 summarizes the recommendations of the Panel on Cost-Effectiveness in Health and Medicine for the correct placement of costs in a cost-effectiveness analysis. It will be much easier to see how different costs and effectiveness measures are incorporated into the cost-effectiveness ratio once we begin working on the sample analysis. We present this information here so that you will be better positioned to understand how cost and effectiveness values are added to the model once you begin to build it.

EXHIBIT 2.1. **Summary Recommendations for the Correct Placement of Costs in a Cost-Effectiveness Analysis**

ACTUAL COSTS INCLUDED IN THE ANALYSIS (NUMERATOR)

- Cost of health care products and services
- Cost of the time a patient spends receiving the intervention
- Cost of travel by the patient and caregivers
- Costs borne by others
- Costs not directly related to health care (for instance, environmental costs)

- Costs associated with mortality
- Costs associated with morbidity
- Costs associated with lost productivity and leisure time
- Cost of time spent recuperating from illness

THEORETICAL COSTS CAPTURED IN THE QUALITY-ADJUSTED LIFE-YEAR (DENOMINATOR)

INTERPRETING THE COST-EFFECTIVENESS RATIO

Let's revisit equation 1.1 from Chapter One yet again:

$$\frac{(\text{Cost of intervention 2} - \text{Cost of intervention 1})}{(\text{Quality-adjusted life expectancy 2} - \text{Quality-adjusted life expectancy 1})} \quad (2.2)$$

Notice that if the incremental cost in the numerator is high but the number of QALYs gained by the intervention is low, the ratio becomes very large. If the cost is high but the number of QALYs is also high, the ratio will be smaller. So you can see that very expensive interventions that are also very effective may still be cost-effective relative to less expensive but less effective interventions.

Researchers do not generally state whether an intervention is cost-effective in medical publications because their area of expertise is research, not policymaking. Instead, it is generally preferred to simply document how the interventions studied compare with other interventions. The most practical strategy for putting the results of an analysis into context is to compare the results of the study at hand to the results of other studies in the same country to provide some basis for comparison (Gold, Siegel, Russell, and Weinstein, 1996). In the United States, the CEA Registry (http://www.tufts-nemc.org/cearegistry/) has simplified this task by presenting cost-effectiveness ratios for many different interventions that comply with the reference case.

FOR EXAMPLE

How Much Does a Drug Really Cost?

Newer cancer drugs such as Avastin cost upward of $100,000 per year (Berenson, 2006). This puts them out of the range of affordability for patients and insurance companies alike. But should such drugs be avoided because of their cost? Cost-effectiveness analysis can be used to indicate how chemotherapy with these drugs compares to chemotherapy without them. If they produce a large number of QALYs, such drugs may well be worth the investment. If they do not, cost-effectiveness analysis can also provide information regarding what one might reasonably pay for the drug. Armed with this information, governments and private insurers can negotiate fair prices with the companies that manufacture the drugs.

EXERCISES 1 AND 2

1. Oseltamivir is a medication that can be used to treat symptomatic infection with the influenza virus (Treanor and others, 2000). (You may have heard about this drug when supplies dried up during the avian influenza scare of 2005–2006.) Doctors know that this drug is effective at shortening both the duration and severity of influenza symptoms, but the medication is expensive and probably not lifesaving when given to youngsters, so the standard of care for treating influenza among healthy adults is to recommend that the person stay home, get some rest, drink plenty of fluids, and have some soup. The cost of not providing the medication can thus be called providing "supportive care" and consists mostly of lost productivity and leisure time.

   Suppose that the average cost of providing oseltamivir to an individual is $100 and the average cost of providing supportive care to an individual is $10. Suppose further that oseltamivir will result in a gain of 0.5 QALYs per person treated and that providing supportive care alone results in a gain of 0.1 QALYs (relative to nothing at all). What is the incremental cost-effectiveness of providing oseltamivir to persons with influenza relative to providing supportive care alone?

2. Suppose that the average cost of vaccinating an individual is $150 and that vaccination results in the gain of 0.75 QALYs per person relative to supportive care. Using information from exercise 1, calculate the incremental cost-effectiveness of influenza vaccination relative to treatment with oseltamivir.

Defining the Comparator

Currently a fraction of the population receives the influenza vaccine at the beginning of influenza season. If we recommend that everyone receive vaccination at the start of the season, this baseline rate of vaccination might increase only a little, because only some people would heed the recommendation. Our incremental cost-effectiveness ratio will therefore be very different if we compare a recommendation for vaccination to current practice than if we compare receiving the vaccination to not receiving it at all.

In the first case, we are talking about a slight increase in the rate of vaccination relative to what is now done. In the second, we are making a much more absolute comparison between doing nothing and giving everyone a vaccination. The comparison intervention is sometimes referred to in economics as a counterfactual.

When comparing interventions, it is important to know how much more or less costly and effective one intervention is relative to what is considered the current standard of care. **Standard of care** refers to that which is generally agreed on to be the best practice. It is also good to know how an intervention stacks up against the **status quo**, or what is actually done in the real world. (Sadly, the standard of care and the status quo are often quite different in medical practice.)

A cost-effectiveness analysis provides the most useful information when it indicates how much more an intervention costs when compared to current medical practice (Gold, Siegel, Russell, and Weinstein, 1996). By including current practice in our analysis, we are calculating a meaningful baseline cost and baseline effectiveness against which we can evaluate the real-world effects of our intervention (for example, the effect of a recommendation for vaccination relative to the current vaccination rates in the population).

It is also helpful to include a "no-intervention" or "do-nothing" comparator. A no-intervention comparator will provide the consumer the cost-effectiveness analysis with a concrete point of reference (Gold, Siegel, Russell, and Weinstein, 1996). If we are to build a league table of incremental cost-effectiveness ratios for setting funding priorities, each ratio must represent the incremental cost-effectiveness of an intervention relative to a common denominator. Because league tables include many interventions that represent the current practice or standard of care, a no-intervention comparator proves to be a useful baseline.

EXERCISE 3

3. What is the policy relevance of a research question focusing on vaccinating everyone in the general population?

Finally, we may wish to know how the incremental cost-effectiveness of vaccination or treatment compares to other interventions that might realistically be used to treat or prevent influenza. Although cost-effectiveness analyses should ideally compare all realistic alternatives to the current standard of care, this is not always possible. At a minimum, the reference case suggests that the most realistic alternatives to the current standard of care should be examined (Gold, Siegel, Russell, and Weinstein, 1996).

TABLE 2.3. **Decision Matrix for Various Cost-Effectiveness Scenarios**

Cost	Effectiveness	Label	Decision
Lower	Higher	Dominant	Implement
Lower	Lower		Decide
Higher	Higher		Decide
Higher	Lower	Dominated	Do not implement

Interpreting Incremental Changes in Cost and Effectiveness

If one intervention is more effective and less expensive than another and the intervention is ethically and socially acceptable, there should be no question that the more cost-effective intervention is preferable. Usually, though, interventions that are more effective are also more costly than the standard of care. When this occurs, the consumer of the cost-effectiveness analysis must decide whether the added effectiveness is worth the added cost.

If a particular intervention is going to cost us money but will improve health, we have to decide whether we are willing to pay the price. If the intervention is going to save money and improve health, it is clear that it's worth doing as long as it doesn't produce any ethical dilemmas and is generally acceptable. In this case an intervention is said to be **dominant** (Drummond, O'Brien, Stoddart, and Torrance, 2005; Gold, Siegel, Russell, and Weinstein, 1996). (See Table 2.3.) If the intervention is more expensive and less effective than the comparator, it is said to be **dominated**. (Whoever said cost-effectiveness researchers were a boring lot?)

TYPES OF ECONOMIC ANALYSIS

Most people are familiar with the term *cost-benefit analysis,* but few can concretely describe the differences between a cost-effectiveness analysis and a cost-benefit analysis. In this section, you will learn how cost-effectiveness analysis differs from the other types of economic analyses and about the related field of burden of disease analysis. Other types of economic analyses complement cost-effectiveness analysis because they provide policymakers and clinicians with different types of information.

Cost-Effectiveness and Cost-Utility Analysis

Although the terms are often used interchangeably (as is the case in this book), health economists distinguish **cost-utility analysis** from cost-effectiveness analysis. From a practical standpoint, a cost-utility analysis can be considered a specific type of cost-effectiveness analysis in which some quality-of-life measure is included in the analysis. A **cost-effectiveness analysis** is a more general term for an analysis that compares the relationship between costs and any outcomes. For example, a cost-effectiveness analysis might compare the cost per number of hospitalizations avoided, cost per number of life years gained, or cost per number of vaccine-preventable illnesses averted. Cost-effectiveness analyses may or may not include a quality measure.

There are also a number of ways in which quality measures, such as HRQL scores, are combined with quantity measures, such as the number of years of life gained by an intervention. Together these measures of quantity and quality fall under the generic category of health-adjusted life years (HALYs), which include QALYs, disability-adjusted life years (DALYs), and healthy-years equivalent (HYE), among others. The reference case analysis uses the QALY (Gold, Siegel, Russell, and Weinstein, 1996).

So what's the difference among these types of HALYs? It mostly comes down to how health-related quality of life is measured. You'll learn about this in Chapter Seven.

When to Use Nonreference Case Cost-Effectiveness Analyses

We have already looked at examples of how deep a health department might go in conducting a cost-effectiveness analysis of tuberculosis treatment strategies. Let's revisit that idea using a different example. Suppose a health department was interested in knowing how many vaccine-preventable diseases could be averted if a vaccine campaign were initiated. By definition, the relevant outcome in this analysis would be the cost per illness averted. A full reference case cost-effectiveness analysis would provide information regarding the effect the vaccine would have on the quality of life of everyone vaccinated and would include costs to employers and other segments of society. However, these outcomes are not relevant to the research question posed by the health department in this example. Nonreference case analyses are generally easier to complete because they require less information, and they may be more useful in circumstances where there is only one relevant outcome.

If a student wishes to conduct a cost-effectiveness analysis that does not incorporate quality-of-life measures using the societal perspective, special considerations must be made. If the outcome of interest is the number of years of life lost to disease, morbidity costs (pain and suffering) are counted in the numerator. The reason is that the HRQL score that theoretically incorporates a subjective measure of these costs is excluded. Students who wish to conduct this type of analysis can otherwise follow the procedures outlined in this book.

If the study is conducted from a specific perspective or includes other measures in the denominator, such as "hospitalizations averted," the costs included and the end points of the study must be carefully thought through. The following exercises should help guide you.

EXERCISES 4 AND 5

4. You are working for a pharmaceutical company that wishes to examine the cost per illness averted for its new human papilloma virus vaccine from the perspective of an insurance company. What morbidity costs do you include?

5. Your boss at La Mega pharmaceutical corporation wishes to add some pizzazz to marketing for a powerful new antibiotic the company developed. She feels that the public won't understand QALYs, so she asks you to present the results of the study in life years gained. Where do you count costs specific to the time a patient spends ill with the disease?

Other Measures

The DALY is frequently used for studies in developing countries and might serve as an international standard for cost-effectiveness analyses (Murray and Lopez, 1996). It may also be used to study immigrants to industrialized nations (Muennig, Pallin, Sell, and Chan, 1999). Unfortunately, there are technical problems with this measure that limit its usefulness and render it incompatible with the reference case scenario (Gold, Siegel, Russell, and Weinstein, 1996; Muennig and Gold, 2001). Students wishing to use the DALY may follow all of the procedures outlined in this book and simply use the HRQL scores tabulated for DALYs by Murray and Lopez (1996). (For technical reasons, DALY scores must be subtracted from 1.0 before they can be used. See Chapter Eight.) The HYE falls to the other extreme. Although it is highly regarded from a technical standpoint, it is difficult to use and might not be an appropriate measure for low-budget studies, such as those conducted in developing countries. For these reasons, the use of quality-of-life measures other than the QALY will be discussed only briefly in this book in the context of cost-effectiveness analysis.

Cost-Benefit Analysis

An alternative to cost-effectiveness analysis that economists sometimes favor is cost-benefit analysis. In this type of analysis, a dollar value is placed on both the costs and the effectiveness of an intervention. In a cost-benefit analysis, all costs are considered, even the intangible costs associated with the disease. The final outcome is reported as a monetary value. Any intervention associated with cost savings (a net benefit) should be undertaken, and any intervention associated with (excess) costs should not. Why? Because everything is properly accounted for, including the amount people are willing to pay to get rid of the disease. Therefore, any treatment with a cost greater than $0 means that the treatment costs more than it's worth.

Some economists argue that cost-benefit analysis is preferable to cost-effectiveness analysis because it produces a more definitive endpoint. Moreover, it is universal. Since cost-effectiveness is mostly used in health and education, we often can't compare investments in medical care to other health investments, such as freeway safety improvements, without conducting entirely new analyses. However, a cost-benefit analysis requires that disease and suffering be valued. Some argue that it is so difficult to place a dollar value on human life and human suffering that most cost-benefit analyses will produce inconclusive results (Gyrd-Hansen, 2005). For instance, the value of a QALY has been estimated to fall between $33,000 and $570,000 (Hirth and others, 2000). Therefore, a cost-benefit analysis of a treatment that produces one additional QALY must have a net cost below $30,000 in order to be relatively certain that it is cost-beneficial. If we stuck to that standard, we would be doing a lot less in health care than we are now.

Cost-effectiveness analyses compare the cost of things of which we can be relatively certain (medications, hospital care, and the like) relative to other outcomes of which we can be relatively certain (QALYs). While estimating health-related quality of life scores is as much art as it is science, QALYs are very good at ranking diseases (Gold and Muennig, 2002). By separating the number of QALYs gained from an intervention from monetary costs, cost-effectiveness analyses avoid the thorny issue of assigning a monetary value to human life.

However, there are few things that we do in modern industrial societies that do not have some impact on health or life expectancy (Tengs, 1995). Factory smog control devices, highway construction, dams, and schools are all examples of things that may have dramatic effects on the health of the communities. For example, although the construction of a dam may be beneficial in reducing air pollution, it may also lead to the displacement of people and communities, affect fish populations, contribute to outbreaks of waterborne infectious diseases, or break and flood towns downstream. And cost-benefit analysis is the tool most often used to evaluate whether such projects should be implemented. Thus, whenever human life is affected in a significant way, a cost-benefit analysis may produce uncertain results.

FOR EXAMPLE

Your Money or Your Life

To convert a cost-effectiveness analysis into a cost-benefit analysis, some researchers have proposed merely placing a monetary value on QALYs and adding this value to the numerator costs of a cost-effectiveness ratio. While many feel that QALYs cannot be valued, there is no shortage of researchers willing to try. In a meta-analysis of the literature to the year 2000, Hirth and others (2000) found that the 1997 valuation of QALYs fell between $25,000 and $428,000 depending on the economic method used to valuate QALYs. (This amounts to $33,000 and $570,000 in constant 2007 U.S. dollars.) Based on a review of the literature and considerations of the value of a statistical life, the U.S. Food and Drug Administration (1999) uses a valuation of $100,000/QALY, or $127,000 in constant 2007 dollars.

Cost-Minimization Analysis

Cost-minimization analysis is useful in cases when the outcome of two interventions is similar but the costs are different (Drummond, O'Brien, Stoddart, and Torrance, 2005). For example, patients with bacterial endocarditis (an infection of the heart) often require long-term treatment with intravenous antibiotics. Traditionally patients with endocarditis were hospitalized while they received therapy. Today antibiotics are sometimes administered at home, potentially reducing the costs associated with this treatment. Because both therapies are equally effective, the only relevant medical issue in evaluating each treatment is the overall cost of administering the treatment at home versus at the hospital. In this situation, a cost-minimization analysis can be used to determine the least costly treatment. Because cost-minimization analysis is easier to conduct than full cost-effectiveness analysis, it should be used whenever two or more interventions of equal effectiveness are being compared.

Burden-of-Disease Analysis

Burden-of-disease analyses do not incorporate information on the cost of a disease. Rather, they are used to determine which diseases are responsible for the most morbidity and mortality within a country and are sometimes used by governments or nongovernmental organizations to allocate health resources.

Traditionally the burden of a disease was measured by the number of years of life lost to that particular disease. Using that definition, diseases with high mortality rates, like malaria and tuberculosis, were thought to be the most significant health problems in the world. More recently, the World Health Organization, the World Bank, and Harvard University redefined burden-of-disease analyses by incorporating a measure of quality of life, the disability-adjusted life-year (DALY), into their definition (Murray and Lopez, 1996). Once quality of life was included, depression, which previously ranked near the bottom of the list, moved up to become one of the world's most significant health problems.

The DALY is a controversial but methodologically solid measure. It's solid because it uses a standard life expectancy value and straightforward calculations that can be fairly and easily applied across countries. It is controversial because of the way HRQL is measured.

Because people of different nationalities and cultures have different perceptions of human suffering and quality of life, the limitations in generating the health-related quality of life scores are exaggerated when conducting cross-national comparisons. To get around this limitation and simplify the collection of HRQL scores, quality of life is measured using the input of experts rather than people residing in a specific culture (Murray and Lopez, 1996). For reasons that will be discussed in Chapter Seven, this renders the DALY incompatible with the reference case scenario of a cost-effectiveness analysis (Gold, Siegel, Russell, and Weinstein, 1996).

One promising alternative to the DALY's HRQL component is the EuroQol, a QALY-compatible measure that has been applied to a growing number of nations (Rabin and de Charro, 2001; EuroQol Group, 1990). For instance, the EuroQol has been included in the Medical Expenditure Panel Survey in the United States, so the burden of disease can be calculated for just about any demographic group, any illness, and many risk factors (Muennig and others, 2005).

CHAPTER

3

DEVELOPING A RESEARCH PROJECT

OVERVIEW

THIS CHAPTER explains how to develop a cost-effectiveness research project. We explore some of the key things to think about as you develop your question, and then go into how to sketch out your model so that you have some idea of what data you'll need to collect.

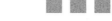

EIGHT STEPS TO A PERFECT RESEARCH PROJECT

Cost-effectiveness analyses are conducted using a series of intuitive methodological steps, many of which may be generalized to any scientific research project:

1. Think through your research question.

2. Sketch out the analysis.

3. Collect data for your model.

4. Adjust data.

5. Build your model.

6. Run and test the model.

7. Conduct sensitivity analysis.

8. Write it up.

9. Have a cup of tea.

   In this book, you'll walk through these steps while looking at applied sample cost-effectiveness analyses. I'll periodically remind you where you are with a project map outlining these eight steps.

   Let us briefly review each step:

1. Think through your research question. A research question is a well-defined statement about your hypothesis on a particular subject or topic. To test your hypothesis, you must clearly indicate which interventions you will be comparing, which subjects you plan to include, and how your analysis will be conducted.

2. Sketch out the analysis. In designing a cost-effectiveness analysis, a researcher must thoroughly review the background information on the disease and health interventions under study (often using clinical practice guidelines) and then chart out the different twists and turns a disease might take when different health interventions are applied. This usually requires sketching out a model on paper.

3. Collect data for your model. Data relevant to your analysis may come from published studies, electronic databases, or other sources, such as medical experts.

4. Adjust your data. Few data will be in a form ready for use in your analysis. For instance, some students will be surprised to learn that the amount providers charge for their services is much higher than the amount the providers are actually paid. Therefore, cost data often need to be adjusted to better reflect real-world costs. Similarly, both cost and probability data often need to be adjusted in such a way that they better reflect the demographic profile of your study cohort.

5. Build your decision analysis model. This model sometimes takes the form of a graphical representation of how your analysis will unfold. It indicates the chances that subjects will see a doctor, receive a laboratory test, and so forth. It also includes the costs associated with each of these events. When run, it melds this information and produces an incremental cost-effectiveness ratio. Fortunately, it is now possible to easily build decision analysis models using basic and intuitive software packages.

6. Run and test your decision analysis model. Before you can be confident that the information your model provides you is accurate, you will need to run some tests. Fortunately, these are usually quite easy to run.

7. Conduct a sensitivity analysis. No data are entirely free of error. A **sensitivity analysis** will evaluate how the error in your data might affect the cost or effectiveness of each of the medical interventions you are studying.

8. Prepare the study results for publication or presentation. Once you have finished your study, you will need to present it in a way that anyone can understand. Adopting standard publication formats helps you achieve this goal (and get published).

DEVELOPING A RESEARCH QUESTION

This section looks at the ins and outs of developing a research question for cost-effectiveness analyses. One of the biggest mistakes beginning researchers make is to think of the comparison they wish to make as a complete research question. This can lead to a lot of unnecessary work. By thinking hard about the characteristics of the groups she or he is comparing, for instance, a beginning researcher will avoid collecting the wrong types of data. The section ends with a research checklist to ensure you have proper footing before embarking on a project.

Anatomy of a Research Question

Every research question in cost-effectiveness analysis should have three key components: (1) information about the population you are studying, (2) a clear description of the interventions being compared, and (3) a definition of the disease you are studying. When broken down into these basic components, the research question naturally presents itself to both the reader and the researcher.

Defining the Population   Cost-effectiveness analyses usually analyze study outcomes for a hypothetical cohort, or a cohort of defined characteristics using multiple sources of data. Suppose we want to know whether it is a good idea to vaccinate all healthy adults against influenza or forgo vaccination in this population altogether. We must first think through what we mean by "healthy." The influenza vaccine is currently recommended for people with chronic lung disease, diabetes, and heart disease, among other conditions (Advisory Committee on Immunization Practices, 2004). Although it may sound crazy, we would still call someone with two broken legs "healthy" as long as he or she didn't have any of the conditions for which vaccination is recommended.

We should also think of the usual demographic characteristics of the population to which we will recommend the vaccine. The most important consideration is age. In this case, we are shooting for people who are over the age of fifteen but under the age of sixty-five. We should also consider whether to include children. Other considerations are income (poor populations are more likely to have most diseases) and gender (some diseases are more common in one gender than another). All of the studies that you find in the literature should come close to matching the demographic profile of the cohort you are defining in your analysis.

Defining the Interventions Under Study   Some students might be thinking, "If healthy adults are already getting vaccinated, what do we mean when we say that we recommend vaccination?" If you are one of these students, you are on your way to becoming a great research scientist. Two critical questions naturally arise from this: (1) Can we reasonably vaccinate everyone in the real world? (2) If not, how many more people are we going to vaccinate above and beyond the number who are now getting vaccinated?

We could "recommend" vaccination for healthy adults, but in most countries this might lead to only a slight increase in current rates of vaccination. Another alternative is to require influenza vaccinations in schools, the workplace, and doctors' offices. This might push the vaccination rates higher still. Alternatively, we could simply evaluate the effect of vaccinating everyone. Although it isn't reasonable to expect that this would really happen in a democracy, it is conceivable that if enough people were vaccinated, transmission of the virus would grind to a halt. This phenomenon, known as "herd immunity," occurs once a critical tipping point of vaccination is reached, say, 70 percent of the population (Advisory Committee on Immunization Practices, 2004).

The next question that naturally arises is: Relative to what? We might compare vaccinating everyone to the current baseline rates of vaccination in the population, or we might compare vaccinating everyone to no vaccination.

For the comparators in which some or all subjects go without a vaccine, we must consider what treatment they do get. Unvaccinated people usually get chicken soup when they get the flu. (Some students might choose tofu soup and echinacea.) They also send their loved ones out to the drugstore to buy some medicine that might make them feel better but won't make them recover any faster.

Let's consider one more example. Suppose that you have been asked to evaluate a new antibiotic against community-acquired pneumonia (as opposed to more dangerous forms of pneumonia one might contract in the hospital). You might compare it against not giving an antibiotic at all, against the most commonly used antibiotic, against the preferred antibiotic (which, sadly, is not the most commonly used), or against "usual care."

Recall that "usual care" or "current practice" implies that interventions are being compared to a mixture of medical interventions that reflect the current practice standards (Gold, Siegel, Russell, and Weinstein, 1996). Therefore, usual care might include some combination of treatments (including inappropriate treatments) that we see in everyday medical practice. If we compare the new antibiotic to usual care, we may be deceiving the consumer of your study. Why? Because "usual care" for pneumonia includes misdiagnoses, the use of inappropriate or expensive medications, or other modalities that are either unnecessarily expensive or ineffective. Such a comparator will make the new antibiotic seem unduly effective since you are comparing it to something suboptimal.

Nevertheless, usual care can be a useful comparator in many cases. For instance, with usual care as the comparator, we can provide policymakers with concrete information about the cost-effectiveness of a campaign that is expected to increase influenza vaccination by 10 percent over the current (usual care) baseline.

Finally, remember that any reference case cost-effectiveness analysis should include a do-nothing comparator that compares the intervention to the natural history of disease (Gold, Siegel, Russell, and Weinstein, 1996). This allows interventions to be stacked up against one another in a league table.

EXERCISE 1

1. You are a policymaker in the Netherlands and wish to know whether it would be a good idea to add a new antibiotic to the drug formulary for community-acquired pneumonia. Currently clinicians use a variety of antibiotics to treat community-acquired pneumonia, but you have the power to change practice patterns. Do you want to know how the new drug compares against the variety of drugs currently prescribed or against what is currently thought to be the best antibiotic?

Defining the Disease You Are Studying Usually, but not always, this part is straightforward. For instance, influenza-like illness is a cluster of diseases that produce symptoms similar to those people have when they are infected with the influenza virus. These symptoms may be induced by the virus itself or by a number of other respiratory tract viruses or bacteria. The World Health Organization defines influenza-like illness as the presence of fever (over 100°F) plus a sore throat or cough (Kendal, Pereria, and Skehel, 1982). Basically, when we have a cold, feel especially lousy, and have a fever, we say we have the "flu." Alternatively, you might use a stricter definition and call the disease "influenza" only when the presence of the virus has been confirmed by a laboratory test.

Our research question might take the form: "Among healthy adults, should we prevent the infection with vaccination, treat flu infections when they arise, or provide supportive care alone?" It sounds pretty good, but there are still a number of things to consider before we continue.

Research Checklist

When you cook lasagna, you know roughly what you'll need to buy at the grocery store, but if you go without a shopping list, you are bound to forget something important. The same is true with scientific research. Therefore, I provide a sample shopping list for any cost-effectiveness research project.

Most books on cost-effectiveness analysis have a checklist against which you can evaluate your research question or, conversely, the research project of others (Drummond, O'Brien, Stoddart, and Torrance, 2005; Gold, Siegel, Russell, and Weinstein, 1996; Haddix, Teutsch, Shaffer, and Dunet, 1996). I've compiled some of the more important points and added a few of my own.

Have I Included All of the Important Alternatives? When considering treatment options, we could include the anti-influenza medications in our analysis, such as oseltamivir. We could compare different doses of oseltamivir or include the inhaled cousin of oseltamivir, called zanamivir (Monto and others, 1999).

In an ideal situation, all comparisons for which uncertainty exists would be included in a cost-effectiveness analysis. The reference case scenario recommends that the standard of care be included as a comparator (Gold, Siegel, Russell, and Weinstein, 1996). It also suggests that the next best alternative to the intervention under study and a no-intervention strategy be included.

Where Will the Intervention Take Place? It is sometimes important to consider the place where a patient will receive the interventions you are studying. For example, if patients are to go to their doctor specifically for a vaccination, the cost of vaccination will be higher than if patients are vaccinated at their workplace. Not only are doctors' offices expensive places to get vaccinated, but you have to drive to get there. Moreover, the total time the recipient spends receiving the vaccine is much higher if he or she has to go to a doctor's office. Not only does one have to drive to get there, but there is also usually a wait. As we say, "Time is money." Therefore, the strategy of vaccinating in the workplace is likely going to cost less than making a special trip to the doctor for the vaccination.

Are Different Levels of Treatment or Different Screening Intervals Relevant? Preventive interventions, such as screening mammography, must often be repeated throughout the patient's lifetime. But how frequently should this occur? If screening tests are performed frequently, the cost of screening will increase, but the chances of catching the disease early will also increase. Therefore, analyses of screening interventions should usually contain a subanalysis examining the cost of screening at different frequencies (Gold, Siegel, Russell, and Weinstein, 1996).

What Type of Study Is Appropriate? This book focuses only on cost-effectiveness analyses with a strong emphasis on cost-utility analysis (because this is the subtype of cost-effectiveness analysis recommended by the Panel on Cost-Effectiveness in Health and Medicine). Nevertheless, keep in mind other ways of evaluating health interventions, such as through a cost-benefit analysis (Drummond, O'Brien, Stoddart, and Torrance, 2005; Gold, Siegel, Russell, and Weinstein, 1996; Haddix, Teutsch, Shaffer, and Dunet, 1996).

If the study is intended for an internal review within a company or government agency but not for publication, then there is less need for a reference case analysis. This relates to the next point: whom you conduct the study for determines how you conduct the study.

For Whom Will I Conduct the Study? The audience of the study determines which costs and outcomes are to be included. For example, when conducting a cost-effectiveness analysis, an insurance company may be concerned only with how much money it will have to spend and how much it might save on a treatment or preventive intervention. It is unlikely that the insurance company will be very interested in whether a patient has to spend money on gas or take a taxi to get to the hospital for a preventive intervention. The audience of the study therefore also determines the perspective of the analysis (Drummond, O'Brien, Stoddart, and Torrance, 2005; Gold,

Siegel, Russell, and Weinstein, 1996; Haddix, Teutsch, Shaffer, and Dunet, 1996). (Remember that the reference case always uses the societal perspective.)

How Far into the Future Do I Need to Capture Outcomes? The **analytical horizon** is the period over which all costs and outcomes are considered (Haddix, Teutsch, Shaffer, and Dunet, 1996). In the case of influenza, a person is ill for a short period of time and then recovers. In the case of adult-onset diabetes, the disease usually arises in middle age and sticks around until death. Therefore, the analytical horizon of the analysis might be the mean age of onset to death.

What Do I Include, and What Do I Ignore? Let's assume for a moment that vaccination saves the occasional life of healthy adults. Thirty-year-old people who die today from influenza might have otherwise lived to be seventy-five, so we might count each year of future life lost in the denominator of our cost-effectiveness ratio. However, these deaths are so rare that they will hardly put a dent in the life expectancy of all healthy adults in our hypothetical cohort.

If you don't count these deaths, the analytical horizon is about five to ten days (the duration of the flu). Excluding deaths therefore greatly simplifies the analysis. If you do count these deaths, we have to account for future years of life lost, and the analytical horizon is human life expectancy.

When a cost makes a dent in the incremental cost-effectiveness ratio, it is said to be "relevant." There is no point in including model inputs that are not likely to make a difference in the incremental cost-effectiveness of a given strategy, but determining what is relevant or not can be challenging.

Ultimately deciding what to include and what to exclude should be part of the agenda of your research team. Model inputs should never be excluded simply because they are difficult or impossible to capture, however (Gold, Siegel, Russell, and Weinstein, 1996). Instead, some attempt at deriving a rough estimate is necessary.

Are There Enough Data to Answer My Question? Some cost-effectiveness analysis questions are not possible to answer because the data are unavailable. Cost-effectiveness analyses may use data from electronic databases, the medical literature, ongoing studies, or even expert opinion. When one key data element is missing, it is possible to conduct a **threshold analysis**. A threshold analysis tells how the results would differ under various guesses surrounding the value of a given parameter. If we did not know how many people become infected with influenza each fall, a threshold analysis would reveal the incidence rate at which vaccination would be the more cost-effective option (Gold, Siegel, Russell, and Weinstein, 1996).

Review

Let's imagine that we have settled on a cost-effectiveness analysis comparing vaccination supportive care. When the time comes for your analysis, you'll scratch similar pertinent information down on a handy piece of paper. It will become crumpled and coffee stained as the months go by, but will serve as your invaluable research partner over the duration of your analysis. Let's take a brief look at what this might look like:

Interventions

- Vaccination required by schools and employers and administered at the worksite or school.

- Assume that vaccine will reduce the incidence of influenza in the general population by 30 percent.

Comparator

- Supportive care is over-the-counter medications plus or minus chicken (or tofu) soup and rest.

Population

- Healthy persons (no chronic lung disease, heart disease, or diabetes) aged fifteen to sixty-five residing in the United States. Also consider secondary transmission to elderly people at risk of complications from influenza (who might benefit from the lower incidence of infection among healthy adults).

Checklist

- All important interventions included? We will not consider oral antiviral medications or laboratory testing for influenza infection.

- Clinical setting? Office, schools, routine medical visits.

- Levels of intervention?

- Vaccination: Mandatory vaccination rather than a recommendation for all employees and school children

- Type of study? Reference case cost-effectiveness analysis.

- For whom? Policymakers.

- Analytical horizon? Life expectancy of cohort.

- What to ignore? Include all possible inputs.

- Are there enough data to answer our question? Yes; however, changes in person-to-person transmission will be difficult to estimate.

DESIGNING YOUR ANALYSIS

Now you have your research question down. The research question is probably the hardest part of an analysis. But once you know what you are about to tackle, it becomes easy to plan your course of attack.

Before you can do that, though, you will need to learn just about all there is to know about the disease. For instance, in the influenza research question, we would need to know the specifics of how influenza is transmitted, how vaccination interrupts transmission of the virus, what the normal course of an infection is, and all of the potential complications of influenza. We will also need information on each of the interventions we are evaluating to prevent or treat it.

Understanding the disease requires reading medical textbooks and review articles. **Clinical practice guidelines** are an important source of information. These guidelines provide perspective on the optimal way to manage a disease in the clinical setting. They are especially helpful because they often contain flowcharts that can be used for inspiration in designing a decision analysis model. One good place to obtain clinical practice guidelines is through the Agency for Health Research and Quality (available at http://www.ahrq.gov). Clinical practice guidelines can also sometimes be downloaded from medical societies such as the American Cancer Society or using a search engine.

Once you have the clinical practice guidelines and other information about the disease in hand, you can chart out the course of the disease when different interventions are applied.

PROJECT MAP

1. **Think through your research question.**
2. *Sketch out the analysis.*
3. **Collect data for your model.**
4. **Adjust data.**
5. **Build your model.**
6. **Run and test the model.**
7. **Conduct sensitivity analysis.**
8. **Write it up.**

The information you'll need to conduct your analysis will probably include incidence rates, mortality data, and costs. These data are obtained from the medical literature, electronic datasets, and other sources. But how do you know exactly what you'll need and where to start? Most people think visually. Therefore, sketching out a chart of events that occur before and after an intervention will provide a framework for your analysis.

Let's again turn to the influenza vaccination example for ideas about how we might approach this question. Figure 3.1 shows one approach to sketching out the

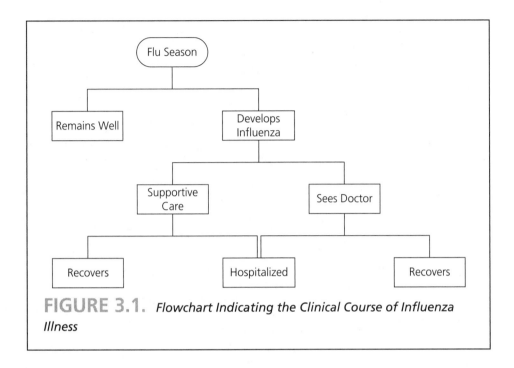

FIGURE 3.1. *Flowchart Indicating the Clinical Course of Influenza Illness*

course of possible events related to influenza virus infection over the typical flu season.

Why is it possible to develop influenza even if you are vaccinated? In reality, the influenza vaccine isn't 100 percent effective in 100 percent of the people who receive it. The scientists who make the vaccine must try to make an educated guess at which strains of the virus will be circulating during the influenza season. They are sometimes only partly right at guessing. Some years they miss altogether, and the vaccine does no good at all. Figure 3.2 charts out the course of the flu among those who receive a vaccination.

In addition to the fact that the influenza vaccination is not always perfectly matched to the vaccine, some people's immune systems do not make antibodies to the vaccine. In other cases, the vaccine helps the body recognize the live virus, but the person develops a mild illness nonetheless. Most vaccinated people are never aware that they were exposed to the virus at all and develop few symptoms. But the point is that the vaccine will never prevent infection in all the people all the time.

In Figure 3.2, the supportive care tree has been removed for simplicity. Here, we see that the vaccine prevents infection in some people (Works) but does not in others (Fails). For those who develop an influenza-like illness despite vaccination, they are less likely to need to see a doctor, less likely to be hospitalized, and less likely to die than those who receive supportive care alone.

Figure 3.2 is an example of an *event pathway*. An event pathway depicts the course of different events that can occur in a cost-effectiveness analysis. Once each of these

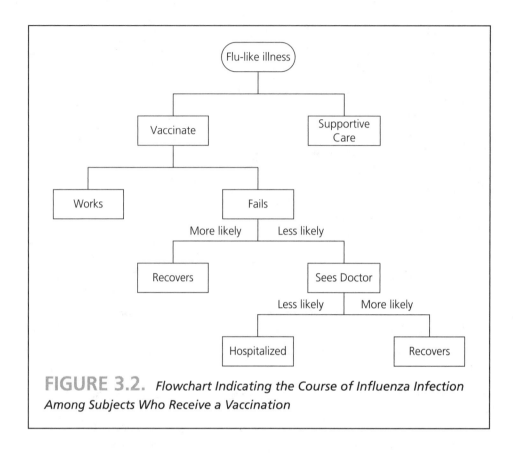

FIGURE 3.2. *Flowchart Indicating the Course of Influenza Infection Among Subjects Who Receive a Vaccination*

events is charted out, you will have a much better idea of which data elements you will need to collect for your analysis. For instance, Figure 3.2 helps us see that those who receive the vaccine are more likely to recover once infected with the influenza virus.

Given that vaccinated people are more likely to recover even if they are infected and become symptomatic, we will need a separate set of probabilities in our event pathway for vaccinated and unvaccinated people (see Figure 3.3). For instance, we need to know the probability that those who developed the flu but received only supportive care will need to see a doctor. We also need to know the probability of a doctor's visit among those who were vaccinated but nonetheless developed the flu. Because this second group has partial immunity to the flu, the probability that they will see a doctor is likely to be lower.

Now let's consider another important probability: the chance that the vaccine will work sufficiently well that those who are exposed to the flu will develop few or no symptoms. This probability, referred to as *vaccine efficacy*, will be a key determinant of how much the vaccination strategy will cost. Let's say that we've gone through the

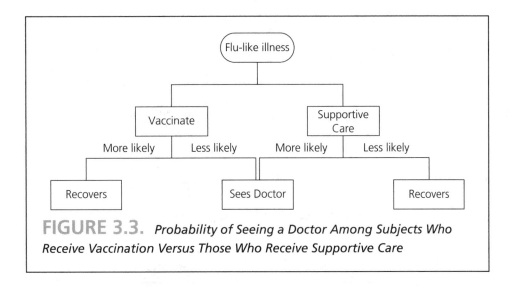

FIGURE 3.3. *Probability of Seeing a Doctor Among Subjects Who Receive Vaccination Versus Those Who Receive Supportive Care*

medical literature and found the vaccine efficacy, the probability of seeing a doctor, and the probability of hospitalization among people who have been vaccinated but who developed the flu anyway (see Figure 3.4).

One key feature of each of these probabilities (seeing a doctor or not, getting hospitalized or not, and so forth) is that they are mutually exclusive events. For instance, you cannot kind of get hospitalized. Moreover, you cannot partially receive a shot for the influenza vaccine (at least not in our model). Therefore, all of the probabilities at any given branch must add up to 1.0. Thus, if we know that the efficacy of the influenza vaccine is 70 percent, the probability of developing the flu despite vaccination must be 100–70 percent, or 30 percent.

Almost all of the "events" (represented as boxes in these figures) in an event pathway are associated with a cost. In Figure 3.4, for example, ill people might see a doctor or might recover on their own. If they see a doctor, they will incur the cost of driving to the doctor, the cost of the doctor's visit, and so on. Sometimes these costs are available in the medical literature, but usually they have to be calculated using a dataset, such as the Medical Expenditure Panel Survey (MEPS). We'll learn how to obtain and adjust these costs in the next chapter.

For now, let's assume that we already have all the costs and probabilities on hand and take a moment to consider how costs and probabilities work together.

Figure 3.5 is a truncated version of the event pathway. Let's call this the "vaccination decision node." (That sounds nice and technical, so it will make all of the academics happy.) Imagine for a moment that we know the cost of vaccine failure ($100 in Figure 3.5). This $100 cost includes the cost of any doctor visits or hospitalizations that occur later, but we'll ignore that for now. The cost of vaccination success is simply the cost of the vaccine ($10, which includes the time to administer it and so forth).

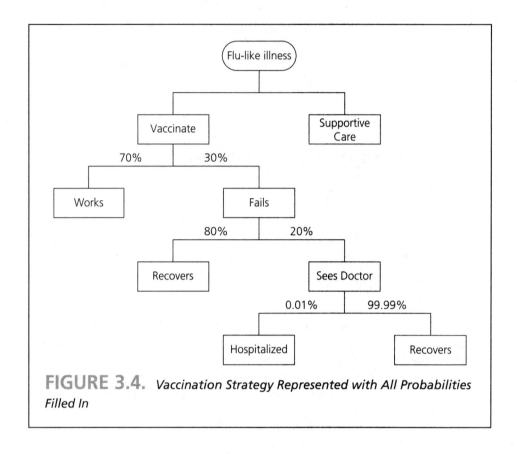

FIGURE 3.4. *Vaccination Strategy Represented with All Probabilities Filled In*

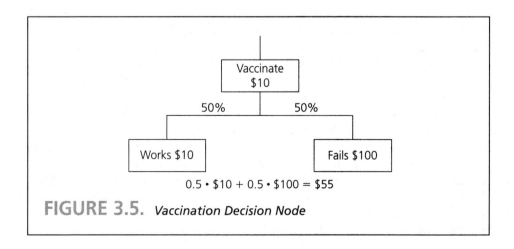

FIGURE 3.5. *Vaccination Decision Node*

Now, let's estimate the overall cost of the vaccination strategy. Pretend that the vaccine was 50 percent effective in the 2006–2007 flu season. We see in Figure 3.5 that our overall cost of vaccination is:

$$0.5 \times \$10 + 0.5 \times \$100 = \$55. \qquad (3.1)$$

It quickly becomes apparent that if we change the vaccine efficacy, our costs will be profoundly affected. For instance, if the vaccine is 70 percent effective during the average season, then the average cost is:

$$0.7 \times \$10 + 0.3 \times \$100 = \$37. \qquad (3.2)$$

Likewise, if the vaccine is 100 percent effective, then the total cost is just the cost of the vaccination, or:

$$1.0 \times \$10 = \$10. \qquad (3.3)$$

So far, you've learned the basics of how to formulate a research question in cost-effectiveness analysis. You've also learned the basics of how costs and probabilities work together. As you will soon see, the effectiveness portion of a cost-effectiveness analysis works in essentially the same way as costs. Before getting into that, let's take a moment in the next chapter to fill in the details of what we've already created and take a deeper look at how costs are actually calculated.

CHAPTER

4

WORKING WITH COSTS

OVERVIEW

SANDRA MONTERO returned to her office after dropping off Sandra Jr. at day care. Sandra always tried to incorporate exercise into her work routine, so after giving the security guard a friendly smile, she turned into the stairwell to make her usual four-flight climb up the stairs, as her doctor recommended. After the first few steps, she felt her thigh muscles ache and suddenly felt tired all over. She lumbered into her office, started to cough, and decided to visit the company physician.

After sitting for almost half an hour in the clinic, the doctor told her that she had the flu. Sandra went home for the rest of the day with instructions to drink plenty of fluids and take some over-the-counter medications. On her way home, she wearily picked up the medicines at a pharmacy near her house, then drove home and climbed in between her fresh linen sheets. Before dozing off, she remembered that Sandra Jr. would soon need a ride home, so she called her baby-sitter and asked him to pick her up from day care.

When Sandra decided to see her physician, she set off a chain of events, each associated with a cost. First, the receptionist, medical assistant, and the doctor each spent time seeing Sandra for her illness. Second, while sitting in the office waiting to see the physician, she unknowingly exposed the receptionist and an elderly file clerk to the influenza virus. The receptionist developed a mild illness that kept her at home for a few days, and the file clerk was eventually hospitalized for bacterial pneumonia that arose as a result of the initial influenza infection. Third, Sandra decided to purchase some over-the-counter medications as recommended by her physician. Fourth, because of her illness, Sandra would stay home from work for the next three days. Finally, the baby-sitter had to leave his other job early to pick up Sandra Jr. from day care.

So you can see how a relatively common illness can translate into a diverse range of medical and nonmedical costs. In our analysis, when thinking about the costs associated with an influenza-like illness, we must take all of these possible events into consideration. Of course, this is just one scenario, and a cost-effectiveness analysis deals with population averages.

In this chapter, we'll take a bit of a break from plotting out and executing our analysis to look at how we might place a monetary value on each of the events Sandra put into motion. You will also learn some of the ways in which costs are collected. More detailed descriptions of how costs are collected can be found in Chapter Twelve.

■ ■ ■

OPPORTUNITY COSTS

Recall from Chapter One that an opportunity cost is the value of goods and services in their best alternative use. If we invest in a mammogram, we are diverting resources from other potentially important investments. When the societal perspective is assumed, goods and services are generally thought of in terms of the social resources that are used rather than prices. By thinking in terms of the resources used when a medical intervention is applied, we will be providing policymakers with better information on whether those resources should be diverted to more efficient projects or interventions.

Although there are many esoteric theoretical reasons for thinking in terms of opportunity costs, there is really one practical reason: in health care, market prices rarely reflect what people actually end up paying. For instance, one gynecologist in New York admitted that he charges uninsured patients $175 for a routine visit but accepts payments of $25 from insurance companies for the same services (Kolata, 2001). The patient walking in off the street is not likely to start bargaining with her gynecologist for a better price. If we were to use the $175 figure in our cost-effectiveness analysis, our estimate would be seven times higher than the standard fee that insurance companies pay.

To estimate the cost of this gynecological visit, we might be better off considering the value of the resources that go into a gynecological visit. For instance, we might place a price on the amount of time the doctor spends with the patient, the number and types of laboratory tests the doctor orders, the overall time the patient spends in the clinic, and the amount the patient spends on transportation to and from the clinic.

FOR EXAMPLE

When to Use Prices

What costs do we include in our analysis when valuing drugs? In theory, the opportunity cost of a drug should include just the manufacturing and distribution costs. Manufacturing costs are difficult to obtain, so cost-effectiveness researchers usually use just the wholesale cost of products (such as drugs). This more practical approach makes sense especially when comparing the cost-effectiveness of pharmaceuticals. Consider two drugs of equal effectiveness with similar manufacturing costs. If one is a brand-name drug and costs twice as much as the other on the market, we would naturally want to purchase the cheaper version. However, an analysis based on manufacturing and distribution costs alone might rate the drugs as equally desirable. A meaningful comparison for policy therefore would require the use of the average wholesale price of one drug versus the other.

We generally use the average wholesale cost of drugs, laboratory tests, and so forth to estimate costs in cost-effectiveness analysis. Why? Because the average wholesale cost is more or less representative of the amount we are paying in the real world and because, for pharmaceuticals, it is the only cost usually available to us. Using the amount that a hospital or doctor bills a patient will distort what is actually paid for such services in the real world. But the use of some opportunity costs can also distort the usefulness of a cost-effectiveness analysis.

Fine. So how do we actually get such information? In the United States, the actual amount paid for a service can be obtained from the Medical Expenditure Panel survey, and the average wholesale price of a drug can be obtained from the *Drug Topics Red Book* (2006). (International data can be found on this book's Web site, http://www.pceo.org, as well as in Chapter Twelve.) When medical expenditures are not available in a given country, it is possible to value the cost of services using wages and the estimated costs of the products consumed. In a moment, we'll go into more detail about how wages and wholesale prices can be used to generate an overall cost. But we should first consider which costs we are actually incurring for a given health intervention.

IDENTIFYING COSTS

In Chapter Three, we saw that vaccination will reduce but not eliminate the likelihood of costly health events. Moreover, people who might never get sick incur the cost of vaccination, so if the incidence of influenza is low, the average cost is high. Recall too that we assumed that the cost of each event in the influenza pathway was essentially the same: whether you've been vaccinated or not, a doctor's visit is still going to set you back $70. However, the probability of incurring a given cost differed depending on the strategy; a vaccinated person is much less likely to get the flu and is therefore less likely to see a doctor.

Since the costs in each pathway are essentially the same, we can merge the vaccination and supportive care strategies when speaking of costs. Figure 4.1 provides a basic framework for identifying the costs that you will use in the analysis. But this is only a basic framework. Within each box, the overall cost comprises a number of smaller costs.

For example, even if she does not see a doctor, Sandra (the subject in the earlier example) will remain at home in bed and will not drive to work while sick. But someone who remains well throughout influenza season will drive to work every day (or take a bus or train). Because the presence or absence of influenza-like illness causes a change in transportation use, the higher rate of transportation among well people could be counted as a cost. Therefore, we might want to change the $0 value in the No Infection box in Figure 4.1.

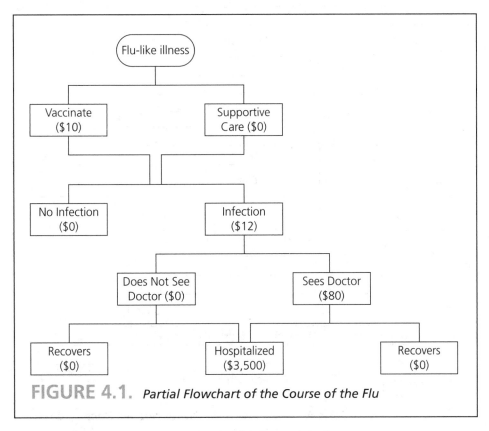

FIGURE 4.1. *Partial Flowchart of the Course of the Flu*

Note: Each box represents a cost associated with influenza infection.

Figure 4.2 provides some examples of the costs associated with the flu even when the subject does not seek medical care. If Sandra stays at home, she is less likely to infect others, which will greatly reduce the overall cost of the supportive care strategy. But she will also miss work, which will partly offset these costs. Don't worry quite yet about how all of these costs are actually captured. Our job for now is to think about

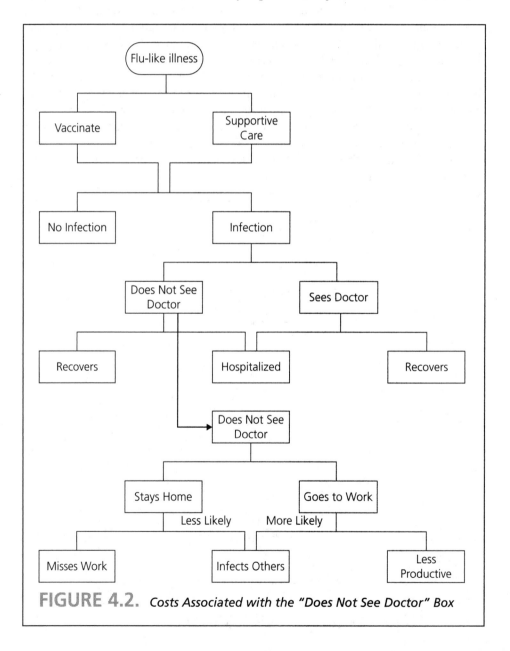

FIGURE 4.2. *Costs Associated with the "Does Not See Doctor" Box*

what types of costs we might consider so that we can make a list of the data elements we will be collecting later on.

Ideally we will want to make a list of costs associated with all of the other boxes as well. Using the overall flowchart as a framework, it is a good idea to break down (identify) all of the costs that lead to the overall cost of each event. This allows us to think more clearly about the subtleties of how costs change when we do something in health or medicine. In practice, though, many of the costs will be obtained in aggregate. For instance, we would probably just look up the average cost of a doctor's visit for influenza virus infection using an electronic dataset.

So why bother with all this business about identifying the resources used? If we do not at least identify all of the costs, we will miss some of the costs that were not included in the value we obtained from an electronic dataset. For instance, the dataset will contain information on the cost of a medical visit but no information about the cost of getting to the doctor in the first place. By identifying all of the minuscule costs involved, we won't miss any important costs.

EXERCISE 1

1. What are some of the costs in the "Hospitalized" box in Figure 4.1 beyond the cost of the hospitalization itself?

MICRO-COSTING AND GROSS COSTING

Costs such as the value of an IV bag or a gallon of gasoline are components of larger costs, such as hospitalization or transportation costs. As such, they are called **micro costs**. Aggregated costs obtained from electronic datasets or from the medical literature are called **gross costs**. The gross cost may not capture all costs in which we are interested. Therefore, it is usually necessary to add some micro costs to gross cost estimates obtained from electronic datasets or the medical literature. Other events in the event pathway may have to be "micro-costed" (in the grammar of health economics) because no gross cost estimates are available.

One example is the cost of the vaccination itself. We are unlikely to find the actual cost of influenza vaccination anywhere in the medical literature or in an electronic dataset. Therefore, we will need to look up the cost of the vaccine, estimate the time a nurse will take to administer the vaccine, estimate the time it will take to receive the vaccine, and consider other costs, such as the cost of a syringe.

So you just learned that the first step in obtaining costs for your cost-effectiveness analysis is to *identify all of the relevant resources that will be consumed* (Gold, Siegel, Russell, and Weinstein, 1996). You also learned that each cost can be obtained by micro-costing or simply using a gross cost. When micro-costing, we need to add two more steps to the process of identification.

Step 2 is to *quantify the resources used.* For example, to estimate Sandra's transportation costs, we might need to know how many miles she lives from her job, how much fuel her car consumes per mile traveled, and so on. This information can often be obtained from census datasets, estimated by expert opinion, or assumed. (Whenever we make an assumption, we must state what the assumption is and why we chose the value we did so that others can judge whether it was reasonable. More on this later.)

Step 3 is to *place a monetary value on the resources used.* The final step in determining a micro cost is to place a monetary value on each resource used. For

TABLE 4.1. **Partial List of Costs for Treatment of Influenza Infection**

Identify	Quantify	Monetize	Total
Nonmedical			
Lost work	5 days	$70/day	$350.00
Patient time	1 hour	$8.75/hour	$8.75
Transportation	10 trips	$1.50/trip	$15.00
Vaccination			
Patient time	0.1 hour	$8.75/hour	$0.88
Medical			
Medical visit			
Receptionist	5 minutes	$0.25/minute	$1.25
Physician	10 minutes	$2.50/minute	$25.00
Vaccination			
Nurse	5 minutes	$0.25/minute	$1.00
Vaccine	8	$2.50/minute	$25.00
Syringe	1	$0.5/syringe	$0.50

instance, we might determine the market price of a gallon of gasoline and multiply this cost by the number of gallons used in driving to work or to the clinic. For patient time costs, wages are applied to the number of hours spent receiving an intervention or treating a patient. Sandra spent thirty minutes at the clinic before the doctor sent her home. If she made $30 per hour, the value of the time spent at the clinic would be 0.5 hours $\times$ $30 = $15.

Now let's take a broader view of the process of identification, quantification, and valuation. Suppose that we were estimating the cost of Sandra's office visit in the example. First, we would identify all of the resources used: the cost of any medical supplies used, any tests performed, Sandra's time, the medical assistant's time, the secretary's time, and the physician's time. To measure the quantity of the resources used, we would estimate the type and number of medical supplies used and the amount of time each person spent treating, or receiving treatment for, the illness. If we were to measure these resources separately, we would assign a wage to each person's time, assign a cost to any tests that might have been performed or supplies used, and then add these costs together. The process of identifying each resource used, measuring these resources, valuing the resources, and adding them together is called **micro-costing**.

Gross costing, using gross costs obtained from a single data source, is generally much easier and less time-consuming than micro-costing, especially when complex hospital costs are involved. It is often possible to obtain a hospital charge for a particular disease in a matter of minutes over the Internet.

Nevertheless, it is easy to overlook important costs when using gross costs. Therefore, we want to make lists of everything, and we need to know whether or not we use micro costs or gross costs. Table 4.1 presents a sample of some of the three-step process discussed above.

GETTING COST DATA

In the previous section, we discussed the process of identification, quantification, and valuation using the example of a medical office visit and vaccination. Suppose we wanted to obtain the cost of the hospitalization (which is what happened to the unlucky elderly file clerk whom Sandra exposed in the waiting room of the doctor's office). The first step, identifying the resources used, would be a huge task.

Micro-costing a hospitalization visit involves accounting for all the gauze pads used, all of the sheets washed, nurse time, and lab services, to name just some of the resources used. If we obtained the cost of hospitalization using a dataset, our efforts would be reduced to looking up the overall cost. This value obtained from a dataset would provide an estimate of all of the medical services used in aggregate. But what have we missed? A few things, as it turns out. For instance, one missing value is the patient's time spent in the hospital.

To measure these additional resources used (beyond the cost of the hospitalization), we need to estimate the patient time cost, which is achieved by obtaining the average length of stay (ALOS) for the hospitalization. The ALOS is an estimate of the time

PROJECT MAP

1. **Think through your research question.**
2. **Sketch out the analysis.**
3. *Collect data for your model.*
4. **Adjust data.**
5. **Build your model.**
6. **Run and test the model.**
7. **Conduct sensitivity analysis.**
8. **Write it up.**

resources used. To assign a monetary value to this resource, we multiply the ALOS by the patient's wage. (We might value the person's leisure time at about the same price as his or her work time, so we can use just the hourly wage for all time costs. For a more detailed discussion, see Gold, Siegel, Russell, and Weinstein, 1996.)

Let's take a moment to see how this works in practice. Give the following exercises a try.

EXERCISES 2 AND 3

2. Obtain the average 2004 hospitalization charge for influenza virus infections. To do so:

   a. Visit http://hcupnet.ahrq.gov/.

   b. Click on "national and regional statistics," and then describe yourself as the elite scientific researcher you are.

   c. Click on "specific diagnoses;" get 2004 data and then ICD-9-specific diagnoses.

   d. Click on "principal diagnosis". You will be asked to enter an "ICD-9 Code." The code for influenza virus infection is: 487. (The "all codes combined" check box should be selected.)

   e. You are after the mean hospital charge, so be sure to check this button and uncheck any others. Notice as you progress through this wizard that you have many alternative options, including patient age. Check the box indicating you are interested in all patients in all hospitals.

3. Assumin-that the average wage is $100 per day, what is the patient's time cost while in the hospital? (Hint: Repeat exercise 2 to obtain mean length of stay.)

If you did exercises 2 and 3, you may have some lingering questions. First, What the did I just do? Second, Is the value that I obtained accurate? We will answer each of these questions in the next two sections. Below, we'll tackle the issue of what you just did. Then we'll tackle how to adjust costs to make sure that they are relatively accurate. For instance, we'll discuss how to adjust the data you downloaded to better reflect its opportunity cost.

TIPS AND TRICKS

Internet links change from time to time. Up-to-date links and exercises can always be found at this book's Web site: http://www.pceo.org.

USING DIAGNOSIS CODES

If you did exercise 2, you conducted a search for all people in the dataset who were hospitalized for influenza virus infection. To ensure that you knew exactly what you were getting, you entered a special code that refers to influenza virus infection. The software pulled all cases within the hospitalization dataset for people diagnosed with influenza virus infection and then provided the relevant information for you in tabular format.

The code that you used is used universally in doctors' offices and hospitals to classify disease. Many students are familiar with these classification systems. If you are one of them, you may skip to the next section.

Diseases are categorized using a number of different systems. These systems include the International Classification for Disease (ICD), Diagnosis-Related Groups (DRGs), and the Clinical Classifications for Health Policy Research, called CCS codes (after the name of the software, the Clinical Classification Software). These codes are generally used to obtain gross cost estimates for medical visits and hospitalizations. Table 4.2 sorts out these acronyms for you.

TABLE 4.2. Common Codes Used to Group Diseases

Classification System	Acronym	Description
International Classification for Disease	ICD	A comprehensive list of every disease and disease subtype
Major Diagnosis Category	MDC	Groups of ICD codes by category (e.g., "Infectious and Parasitic Diseases" or "Neoplasms")
Clinical Classifications for Health Policy Research	CCS	Groups of ICD codes by common diseases and subtypes (for example, diabetes and its various complications)
Diagnosis-Related Groups	DRG	A list of over 500 diseases grouped by costs

The online dataset you used is called the Healthcare Cost and Utilization Project. As you saw in the exercise, you could have used any number of disease classification systems. The ICD system is currently in its tenth revision and is often referred to by its revision number. For example, the ninth revision is still commonly used and is referred to as the ICD-9 system. Costs obtained from this system are specific to a particular disease. For instance, using this system, it is possible to obtain costs for either influenza virus hospitalizations or for pneumonia secondary to influenza. In the ICD-9 system, the codes are five digits. The first three digits refer to the disease in question. For example, conduct disorders use code 312. The last two numbers refer to disease subtypes. For instance, pathological gamblers get code 31231, kleptomaniacs get code 31232, and pyromaniacs get code 31233.

Sometimes this system can be too specific. For example, diabetes mellitus can cause many different complications, each associated with its own ICD code. Examining diseases with a number of different complications takes a lot of effort to figure out which ICD codes go with which diseases. For this reason, it is sometimes preferable to use a less specific system when examining costs associated with complex diseases.

The Clinical Classifications for Health Policy Research system's CCS codes solve this problem. It groups ICD codes specific to a particular disease. For example, CCS codes can be used to examine costs for five ICD codes that are related to diabetes mellitus without complications (CCS code 49) or thirty-eight conditions associated with complications for the disease, such as circulatory, neurological, or kidney problems (CCS code 50). They can also be used to examine each specific complication of the disease. For example, different kidney problems associated with the disease (ICD codes 25040–25043) are grouped together into diagnosis category 3.3.2.

The CCS code for influenza is 123. Take a moment, and compare the charges obtained using an ICD-9 code and a CCS code using the Healthcare Cost and Utilization Project Web site. You'll notice that your mean length of stay and mean charges have changed because we are capturing conditions caused by the influenza virus infection in addition to full-blown influenza infections.

While the CCS system aggregates codes for a particular illness, the DRG system aggregates diseases with similar costs. It is therefore the least disease-specific system. For example, costs related to diabetes mellitus mostly differ by the age of the patient and are listed as "Diabetes, less than age thirty-five" and "Diabetes, greater than age thirty-five." Other endocrine diseases are less common and are similar in cost, so those with an uncomplicated stay in the hospital are grouped together under the general category "Endocrine disorders without complications."

As we will see in a moment, DRGs are useful for adjusting hospital charges obtained from electronic sources.

ADJUSTING COSTS

Costs obtained from the medical literature or electronic datasets often require adjustment before they can be included in a cost-effectiveness analysis. Suppose that you have found a good study on the cost of ambulatory care for influenza-like illness, but the study was conducted in 2000 and your other costs are from 2006. Because prices have inflated since 2000, you can't simply use the earlier cost in your analysis. Whether costs will occur in the future or have occurred in the past, they need to be adjusted to present values. (The net cost of an intervention in present terms is called the **net present value**.)

Other forms of adjustment are also needed. Some costs, such as those you obtained in exercise 2, might be in the correct year but might include huge profits and therefore need to be adjusted to reflect the opportunity cost of the intervention better. Hospital charges are the primary example of this type of cost distortion.

PROJECT MAP

1. **Think through your research question.**
2. **Sketch out the analysis.**
3. **Collect data for your model.**
4. *Adjust data.*
5. **Build your model.**
6. **Run and test the model.**
7. **Conduct sensitivity analysis.**
8. **Write it up.**

Hospital Charges

Data on hospitalization costs are most often obtained from hospital billing systems, which report the total bill—the **charge**—incurred by the patient. A charge is the amount that a hospital, clinic, or pharmacy bills the patient or the patient's insurance company. Some of the goods and services for which hospitals charge are inflated so that the hospital can generate profits or recover losses from investments that are unrelated to the billed admission. For instance, overbilling is one way to cover care provided to uninsured patients. (This is perhaps called "overbilling" because "overcharging" sounds too harsh.) Hospital charges are therefore almost always larger than the actual cost of the resources used. The World Health Organization (2003) reckons that in the United States, actual costs are about 57 percent of the average amount charged.

TIPS AND TRICKS

If you are conducting research in industrialized nations other than the United States, you can skip to the "Adjusting for Inflation" section below.

Charges are relevant only when the free market sets the price of medical care. Thus, they apply only to largely unregulated private insurance schemes, such as those in the United States, China, and India. Private health insurance policies are increasingly available to private purchasers in Europe and Australia as a complement to the national health system. Nonetheless, countries with national health systems typically report government costs in their datasets. They can therefore be used in a cost-effectiveness analysis without adjustment because they generally reflect the cost of the care that the average person uses. Since public sector programs in the United States provide services only to populations that are generally quite demographically different from the rest of the population (the poor, Native Americans, armed forces personnel, the elderly), these government costs tend not to reflect the cost of care for the average person.

This does not mean that government cost data in the United States are not useful. Although the reported Medicare costs apply only to persons over the age of sixty-five or those with debilitating chronic diseases, Medicare costs can be used to generate **cost-to-charge ratios**. These ratios can then be used to adjust any charge obtained from any dataset.

Medicare conducts an extensive analysis of the actual costs of hospitalizing a patient to ensure that it is paying only for the services consumed by its patients. When a Medicare patient is hospitalized, Medicare generally does not pay the hospital what the patient was charged. Rather, it pays the hospital an amount that is roughly equal to the cost of the goods and services the hospital provides to the typical patient with a similar condition.

Medicare cost data are available through a system called Medical Provider Analysis and Review (Medpar). In Medpar, each charge made to Medicare and each payment made by Medicare is listed by DRG (see Table 4.3). A list of cost-to-charge ratios generated using Medicare data can be found in Appendix D. The book's Web site contains links to Medpar data at http://www.pceo.org/cost.html (the direct government link is horrendously long and always changing).

TABLE 4.3. Medpar Cost Data by DRG

DRG	Total Charges (1)	Covered Charges (2)	Medicare Reimbursement (3)	Number of Discharges (4)	Average Days (5)
1	$1,928,498,183	$1,915,759,780	$623,270,066	34,350	9
2	$438,208,550	$435,948,632	$133,227,638	6,906	10
3	...	...	...	...	...
79	$3,153,694,276	$3,120,337,113	$1,323,306,929	171,606	8.5

Notice in Table 4.3 that Medicare lists the amount it was charged (Total Charges), the amount of the charge that is covered (Covered Charges), and the amount it actually paid (Medicare Reimbursement). This last amount is the cost of the services rendered.

By forming a ratio of the reimbursements in column 3 by the charges in column 2 of Table 4.3, you can convert any ICD or CCS code to a cost that will more or less work for any age group or coding system. For instance, if we needed to convert a hospital charge of $10,000 for influenza virus infection to a cost, you might use DRG 79 (the final row in Table 4.3), which is "infectious and inflammatory respiratory conditions with complications." A rough estimate of the opportunity cost of this $10,000 charge is:

$$\frac{\$10,000 \times \$1,323,306,929}{\$3,120,337,113} = \$4,196. \tag{4.1}$$

This ratio is the cost-to-charge ratio. As the name implies, it adjusts hospital charges so that they better reflect the cost of the social resources used when a patient is hospitalized.

We can use the information contained in the Medpar system to estimate cost-to-charge ratios by looking for a DRG that is similar to the ICD-9 or CCS charge we wish to use. Suppose that we wish to know the average cost of hospitalization for pneumococcal pneumonia, a specific type of bacterial pneumonia. We could pull the mean hospitalization charge for this type of pneumonia (ICD-9 code 486) from the health care cost and utilization project Web site, and then adjust the cost according to what Medicare was charged and what it paid for cases of simple pneumonia (DRG 89). Let's give this a try.

EXERCISES 4 AND 5

4. Calculate a cost-to-charge ratio for DRG 89 (simple pneumonia) using Medicare's Medpar data (see Appendix D).

5. Calculate the average hospitalization costs for bacterial pneumonia (ICD-9 code 486) from the Healthcare Cost and Utilization Project (available at http://hcupnet.ahrq.gov/), and convert these into a cost using the cost-to-charge ratio you calculated in exercise 4. Use 2003 data this time rather than 2004 data.

Converting Other Charges

Data specific to national health systems outside the United States are usually presented in the form of costs rather than charges. When data include charges in the private sector, there is little hope of obtaining an accurate cost-to-charge ratio in many countries. Here you may need to consult with experts in insurance companies to obtain estimates of local cost-to-charge ratios. (Typically they've done the footwork to see how little they can get away with paying.)

Most researchers in the United States obtain cost data from the Medical Expenditure Panel Survey (commonly referred to as MEPS and available at http://www.meps.ahrq.

gov/mepsweb/data_stats/MEPSnetHC.jsp). This dataset allows one to obtain charges *or* expenditures for medical visits and has an online tool similar to the Healthcare Cost and Utilization Project used in exercise 2. So, can expenditures be used as a proxy for costs?

Expenditures reflect what the patient or insurance company actually paid for the billed charges. A good deal of care is charitable. Patients who received charitable care will have an expenditure of $0 for their medical visit. Conversely, some people will be "overbilled" for their treatment and pay this large amount. In these instances, the expenditures will be inflated.

One examination of expenditures found that these two factors—free care and inflated charges—just about balance each other out and that expenditures in MEPS serve as a good proxy for costs (Muennig and others, 2005). Of course, since low-income, uninsured populations receive charitable care, they are likely to have many $0 expenditure values. Therefore, any analysis examining low-income groups alone would likely produce an underestimate of real-world expenditure values.

TIPS AND TRICKS

The online tool for MEPS does not yet have the ability to access diseases by diagnosis code, so it is necessary to work with someone familiar with electronic data in order to obtain MEPS expenditures for specific diseases.

Adjusting for Inflation

When older cost data are used, they underestimate the cost of medical care in current terms unless they are adjusted for inflation. The methods section of most research papers states the year in which all costs were obtained, and electronic data-sets always indicate the year for which the data were collected.

TIPS AND TRICKS

The examples presented here are for the United States, but students (or researchers) from any other country can follow along. A search engine should quickly get you to your relevant national consumer price index page.

To inflate older cost data in the United States, visit the U.S. Bureau of Labor Statistics home page (http://www.bls.gov/cpi/home.htm). Under "Latest Numbers," you should see a graphic of a green dinosaur (an icon for all things old). If you click on the little green guy, you get historical cost data. Consumer prices in general (CPI-U for Consumer Price Index for Urban Consumers) are valued differently from medical prices. Medical care prices tend to go up more quickly than consumer prices, so these costs should be inflated independent of consumer costs in any cost-effectiveness analysis.

After clicking on the dinosaur icon on the Bureau of Labor Statistics Web site, you should be presented with a table listing the changes in the price of medical care over the years you requested. The annual changes in medical inflation between 1995 and 2005 for the United States appear in Table 4.4.

TABLE 4.4. **Medical Portion of the Consumer Price Index 1995–2005, Annual Percentage Change on Previous Year**

Year	Percentage Change
1995	4.5
1996	3.5
1997	2.8
1998	3.2
1999	3.5
2000	4.1
2001	4.6
2002	4.7
2003	4
2004	4.4
2005	4.3

TIPS AND TRICKS

If you save tabular data from Web sites with an .htm extension (regardless of your browser or operating system), you should be able to open the table in a spreadsheet program.

It is important to remember that these figures might not apply to a specific treatment or disease. For example, new drugs that were introduced to the U.S. market in 1996 greatly reduced the mortality rates for HIV in developed countries but also had a large impact on the cost of care. Thus, a study on the cost-effectiveness of an intervention to treat HIV that used 1998 data would likely produce a dramatically different result than if data from two years earlier were used. Therefore, simply adjusting these costs for inflation would not suffice.

EXERCISE 6

6. You are conducing a study on a new modality to prevent heart disease but need the cost of a doctor's visit to complete your analysis. You find a study from 2002, but other data you are using are from 2005. Inflate the cost of this $100 ambulatory medical visit in 2002 to 2005 dollars using Table 4.4.

Discounting Future Costs

Medical interventions, especially preventive interventions, often result in decreased future medical costs that must be accounted for in present-day terms. Humans have a tendency to place a lower value on future events than on events that occur in the present. This phenomenon is called **discounting**. For example, if someone were to offer you $100 today or $103 a year from now, you would probably forgo the extra three dollars to have the money in your pocket today.

If you wait for a payment, you may never get it. The person giving out the money might not be able to pay it in a year, or as the receiver, you might die before you have a chance to spend it. Of course, there are other reasons that people wish to have things immediately rather than in the future, one being simple human impatience.

If you were willing to wait one year to receive an extra $3 on an investment of $100, you would earn 3 percent by waiting ($100 × 1.03 per year = $103). Imagine that you were ambivalent about whether to accept $103 a year from now or $100 today. Imagine also that you were certain that you would not be willing to accept either $99 today or $102 a year from now rather than $100 today. If $103 is the minimum amount you'll accept in one year, your time preference is said to be 3 percent (Olsen and Bailey, 1981). **Time preference** refers to the discount rate that a person places on future expenditures.

If $3 is the minimum interest you'll accept, the value of $103 delivered one year into the future is equal to $100 today. This $100 is the net present value, or the value of $103 in future earnings discounted into present terms at a 3 percent rate of discount. By discounting all future costs into their present-day terms, we are accounting for the human tendency to place a lower value on future earnings.

When to Use Discounting

Most cost-effectiveness analyses contain future costs. If a treatment for diabetes or high blood pressure prevents hospitalizations that occur more than one year into the future, these costs should be discounted. In fact, in cost-effectiveness analysis, all future cost and effectiveness values must be discounted into their net present value (Gold, Siegel, Russell, and Weinstein, 1996).

TIPS AND TRICKS

Future QALYs must be discounted in a cost-effectiveness analysis at the same rate as costs (3 percent). The reasons are more practical than theoretical: if we use a different rate of discount in the numerator and the denominator of the incremental cost-effectiveness ratio, discounting will lead to accounting problems.

The Panel on Cost-Effectiveness in Health and Medicine bases the recommended discount rate on a valuation that is roughly equal to the real rate of return on government bonds (Gold, Siegel, Russell, and Weinstein, 1996). Because this rate varies over time and the reference case is concerned with making all cost-effectiveness analyses comparable, the panel has settled on a rate of 3 percent. Although this rate was set to be reevaluated in 2006, no action was taken in that year. One participant predicted that the 3 percent rate would not change for the foreseeable future (J. Lipscomb, personal communication, March 28, 2006).

To maintain comparability with older cost-effectiveness analyses and make sure that the results of studies conducted in the present will still be useful in the future, the Panel on Cost-Effectiveness in Health and Medicine also recommends that the study results be presented with no discount rate applied as well as with a rate of 7 percent (Gold, Siegel, Russell, and Weinstein, 1996).

Internationally, many studies use a discount rate of 5 percent (Drummond, O'Brien, Stoddart, and Torrance, 2005). However, standards vary from country to country.

How to Use Discounting

The general formula for discounting future costs is:

$$\frac{\text{Cost of future event}}{(1 + \text{discount rate})^{\text{years in future}}} \tag{4.2}$$

For example, if the hypertensive person in the example above were to suffer a stroke ten years into the future and was hospitalized at a cost of $10,000, the cost of the hospitalization ten years down the line in present-day terms at the standard discount rate of 3 percent would be:

$$\frac{\$10,000}{(1.03)^{10}} = \$7,441 \tag{4.3}$$

Let us give a more practical example of how this formula is used. Suppose that we find that the average elderly person with high blood pressure has a hospitalization cost of $10,000 per year. If we know that the average person in an elderly cohort will live ten years, the total hospitalization costs and discounted hospitalization costs (at the standard 3 percent rate) might assume the form of Table 4.5.

In Table 4.5, we see that the ten-year total cost comes to around $88,000, or about $12,000 less than it would have had the figures been discounted. As with Table 4.4, this assumes that the first hospitalization charge occurred at the end of the year. Had it occurred at the start of the year, we would have discounted the original $10,000 as well.

TABLE 4.5. Hypothetical and Discounted Costs of a Cohort of 1,000 Elderly Persons over Ten Years

Year	Time (1)	Total Cost Per Person (2)	Discounted Cost (3): Col. 2 /(1.03)^Col. 1
2006	0	$10,000	$10,000
2007	1	$10,000	$9,709
2008	2	$10,000	$9,426
2009	3	$10,000	$9,151
2010	4	$10,000	$8,885
2011	5	$10,000	$8,626
2012	6	$10,000	$8,375
2013	7	$10,000	$8,131
2014	8	$10,000	$7,894
2015	9	$10,000	$7,664
Total			$87,861

The general formula for discounting a cost over many years is:

$$\sum_{1}^{T} \frac{C_y}{1.03^{y-1}} \qquad (4.4)$$

where T is the mean number of years of life remaining in the cohort, and C_y is the cost for year y.

TIPS AND TRICKS

Variations in your start time will affect the estimated future value. For instance, if you find that the cost of hospitalization for tonsillitis in 2007 is $12,000, the future value will vary depending on whether the $12,000 figure was obtained January 1, 2007, or June 1, 2007. If the latter, then the discounted cost on January 1, 2008, would be $12,000/$(1.03)^{0.5}$ = $11,824 rather than $12,000/$(1.03)^{1}$ = $11,650.

COSTS ASSOCIATED WITH PAIN AND SUFFERING

One way to think about the costs associated with pain, suffering (morbidity costs), and death (mortality costs) is that they are intangible. **Intangible costs** are perceived costs that do not have a market value. In the reference case scenario, intangible costs are captured in the HRQL score and are therefore counted in the denominator of the cost-effectiveness ratio.

Costs captured by the HRQL score include those associated with (1) pain and suffering, (2) death, (3) lost productivity, and (4) lost leisure time. We will learn more about how the HRQL score actually captures these costs later. For now, just keep in mind that they are captured in the denominator of a reference case cost-effectiveness analysis. If one were to conduct a cost-benefit analysis or a cost-effectiveness analysis that does not incorporate HRQL scores, these costs have to be estimated.

Of the intangible costs captured by the HRQL score, it's most important to pay attention to lost productivity and leisure time lost to disease. These are examples of costs that are imperfectly captured in the HRQL score. Perhaps more important, they have to be distinguished from the time costs associated with medical treatments.

TIPS AND TRICKS

The Health Utility index, a generic preference-weighted instrument used to generate HRQL scores, explicitly excludes a valuation of lost productivity. When this instrument is used, lost productivity due to illness must be added to the numerator of a cost-effectiveness ratio.

Time costs are those costs associated with the time a patient spends receiving a medical intervention or medical care. Unlike lost productivity, morbidity, or mortality, time costs are included in the numerator of an analysis. These costs are included because HRQL valuations do not capture these costs. (The reasons will be discussed later.) Similarly, if a caregiver or any other person must spend time away from day-to-day activities as a result of the intervention or the disease under study, the time should also be included as a cost.

Time costs are almost always determined using micro-costing techniques, usually by multiplying the time spent in treatment by the mean wage of the subjects under study.

The time in transit to a medical clinic can be found in published cost-effectiveness analyses or assumed. In industrialized nations, time in transit will be different for less serious conditions and diseases than for those requiring specialty medical care. When people in wealthy nations seek specialty care, such as care for cancer, they often want the best possible care available, so many travel long distances to well-known clinics (Secker-Walker and others, 1999).

In developing nations, patient time costs can be quite small because mean wages can be very low relative to the cost of the medical care they receive. Nonetheless, people who live in rural areas may have to travel for days to reach the nearest medical facility. Because data are not usually available in the developing context, costs nearly always have to be estimated. However, locals tend to have a good sense of how long the trip will take. Therefore, a qualitative assessment of travel times by the folks you are evaluating may serve as a good proxy for hard data.

The duration of physician contact by disease and physician specialty is available from the National Ambulatory Medical Care Survey (NAMCS) (Schappert and Nelson, 1999); however, this does not include an estimate of the time a patient spends waiting in the office. The mean contact time with a physician in an ambulatory setting is about nineteen minutes (Schappert and Nelson, 1999).

You calculated the average length of stay in exercise 3. The average length of stay is, of course, a good estimator of the time a patient spends in the hospital.

Practically speaking, the wage that a person earns provides a good estimate of the opportunity cost of a patient's time or a caregiver's time. When the patient is not paid, the wage of an equivalent job may be used. For instance, an unpaid parent's time may be valued at a housekeeper's wage. (For a comprehensive list of earnings by profession, visit http://www.bls.gov/bls/wages.htm.)

Problems arise in valuing a person's time when the study focuses on women or minority populations. African Americans earn less than whites, and women earn less than men. In addition to the fact that the lower wages paid to these groups may not reflect the true opportunity cost of their labor, there is a strong ethical argument to be made that everyone's time be valued equally.

Consider, for instance, valuing the time spent receiving cancer screening. If a homemaker's wage is $8 per hour and an associate in a law firm pulls in $240 per hour, we might find that cancer screening is cost-effective only if administered to homemakers.

In theory, interventions targeted to African Americans or other minority groups or interventions targeted toward women (for example, screening mammography) should be calculated using both average wages and the wages of the group of interest. The difference in the wages between these groups can be seen as a type of systematic error in the way society values human labor, and this error can be tested in a sensitivity analysis. In practice, most researchers use the median wage for a given society and apply it to everyone.

ASSESSING THE "RELEVANCY" OF COST DATA

While it is important to identify all costs included in a cost-effectiveness analysis, we need only measure, valuate, and include those costs that are likely to be relevant to the analysis (Gold, Siegel, Russell, and Weinstein, 1996). But what does *relevant* mean?

In this section, we review some of the important points to consider when evaluating cost data for its relevancy.

Consider Guillain-Barré syndrome, a potentially fatal neurological complication of influenza vaccination. Approximately 1 in 1 million people who receive the vaccine may develop this condition. Of those who develop it, about 6 percent will die (Lasky and others, 1998). Although these numbers are small, it is not clear whether the cost of this condition will be relevant. This syndrome may require extended hospitalization and, in some cases, long-term care. The cost of the Guillain-Barré syndrome, $100,800 (range $70,000 to $130,000), is available from the medical literature (Meltzer, Cox, and Fukuda, 1999, available at http://www.cdc.gov/ncidod/eid/vol5no5/meltzer.htm).

The cost of Guillain-Barré in a cost-effectiveness analysis is, of course, dependent on the probability of incurring the cost. The probability of incurring the cost is 1 in 1 million. Therefore, the total cost will be $0.000001 \times \$100,800 = \$0.10$. If the overall cost of the vaccination strategy is $10, a cost of 10 cents amounts to rounding error.

OTHER COST CONSIDERATIONS

Sometimes it's necessary to evaluate the cost-effectiveness of the way things are done in an institution rather than conduct a simple comparison of diseases. At other times, the cost-effectiveness analysis may have such a large impact on medical care utilization nationwide that one must consider changes in the efficiency of large institutions. Finally, theoretical concerns sometimes arise when a given health intervention produces a marked increase in human life expectancy. In this section, I first discuss a framework for thinking about when costs need to be measured and then look at cost considerations that come up less frequently in cost-effectiveness analysis.

Measuring Changes in Costs

If we are measuring the cost of vaccination at IBM, we don't care what the market value of IBM is; we are concerned only with how much money will be spent on adding a vaccination program. In short, we are concerned only with costs that change as a result of the intervention. Because cost-effectiveness analyses measure changes in costs, it is important to be able to identify which costs change when an intervention is undertaken and which costs do not. In this section, you will learn how to think about the dynamic and static properties of costs.

Costs that change when a medical intervention is applied are referred to as **variable costs**. When Sandra Montero visited the company clinic, she exposed others to the influenza virus. She also took up some of the secretary's time, the medical assistant's time, and the doctor's time. Her decision to visit the company clinic therefore consumed resources that would not otherwise have been consumed, and each of the resources is an example of a variable cost.

Fixed costs are costs that do not change because of a health intervention. Whether Sandra had visited the clinic or had gone directly home, the janitors would have to clean the clinic at the end of the day, the rent has to be paid, and so on. Administration, maintenance, medical equipment, computers, and other things that would have been bought with or without the existence of influenza patients are examples of fixed costs and should generally not be included in the analysis.

Of course, there are exceptions to this rule. Suppose that the company instituted an influenza vaccination policy that resulted in a dramatic drop in patient illnesses and visits to the clinic. The administration might choose to reduce the clinic's hours of operation to compensate for the lighter volume or even to close the clinic altogether. In this instance, the intervention (influenza vaccination) would have had a significant impact on the consumption of resources that might otherwise have been considered "fixed." If an intervention results in sufficient changes in patient volume to cause changes in staffing levels or changes in the wear and tear on medical equipment, or (conversely) merits purchasing new equipment, these changes should be accounted for if they are likely to be relevant for the analysis.

When to Use Micro-Costing

In some hospitals, when a patient comes into the emergency room with a stroke, the doctors must order medications from the hospital pharmacy. The order is often written on the patient's chart and subsequently sent to the pharmacy for review before it is dispensed. Although this sequence of events is generally expedited in emergencies, it can still take considerable time, because the pharmacy may be located in a different part of the hospital.

It is conceivable that by the time the order is completely processed and the medication becomes available in the emergency room, the patient may have suffered serious damage from the stroke. We may therefore wish to evaluate an intervention that improves the way that emergency medications are supplied within the hospital. Since this involves shuffling around micro costs, it is nearly impossible to conduct such an analysis using gross costing methods.

For instance, suppose that the intervention is to simply make these lifesaving medications available in the emergency room. This would greatly reduce the time required to get the medication to the patient. However, when medication dispensing is not tightly regulated and is administered emergently, dosing errors occur more often. Because the pharmacist is not overseeing the transaction, it is also possible that the wrong medication may be administered. A cost-effectiveness analysis examining this issue might assist hospital administrators in deciding whether it is better to keep these medications in the pharmacy or have them available in the emergency room. Clearly, the overall cost of a hospitalization for stroke is going to do very little to help us out with this analysis.

Micro-costing should be used when the cost-effectiveness analysis is centered on changes in the way the resource is delivered. Micro-costing is also useful when a particular cost is not available in the medical literature or electronic data. For example, in our influenza study, we won't have an estimate of the cost of side effects to vaccination, so we will need to micro-cost these events. Micro-costing may also more closely esti-mate the opportunity cost of medical goods and services (Gold, Siegel, Russell, and Weinstein, 1996).

The major disadvantages of micro-costing are that it requires a lot of work, costs can be missed, and the costs you do get often lack **external validity**. External validity refers to the extent to which the results of a study are generalizable to settings other than the one in which the data were collected. For instance, if we obtained the cost of a vaccine from New York City, it might not reflect the cost of a vaccine in Tulsa, Oklahoma. This is especially a problem in analyses using data across developing countries, where the cost of a drug, laboratory test, or medical services can vary by tenfold from one country to another.

Micro-costing is also resource intensive, especially when applied to complex costs, such as the cost of hospitalization. Unless one uses administrative systems designed to measure resource consumption, it is also easy to miss important costs.

Friction Costs and Transfer Payments

Within the context of cost-effectiveness analysis, *friction costs* are incurred when an intervention increases administrative expenses. One example is when absenteeism or unemployment rates increase because of illness. Such costs can usually be excluded from a cost-effectiveness analysis because they tend to be very small relative to other costs. In those rare instances in which an intervention is expected to have a very large impact on administrative costs at a worksite or in a government agency, researchers should consider including friction costs in their analysis (Gold, Siegel, Russell, and Weinstein, 1996).

Transfer payments are payments made from one entity to another as part of a social contract, such as social security payments. For instance, workers pay into the social security system with the expectation that the money will be returned to them when they retire. In this instance, the money is transferred from workers' paychecks to the government and is then transferred back from the government to the worker at a later date. The only resources consumed when transfer payments are made are the fric-tion costs of administering such programs. Therefore, only the friction costs associ-ated with transfer payments need to be included in a cost-effectiveness analysis. And even then, they need to be included only if they will be sufficiently large to merit their inclusion.

Savings Associated with Premature Death

While future medical costs can be reduced by a successful health intervention, they can also be lowered as a result of a premature death. If an intervention is effective at reducing the severity of a disease, then future ambulatory care, hospitalization, and medication costs will all likely be lower among those who received the intervention. However, future medical costs will also be lower if someone dies prematurely from an accident or some other unfortunate event.

Typically such costs are lower than wages, so death is often economically undesirable if it happens to a young person. But if we count savings in future medical costs for someone who dies around the age of retirement, it can seem as if death is desirable from an economic standpoint ("Epidemics and Economics," 2003; Gold, Siegel, Russell, and Weinstein, 1996). For example, one study found that smokers actually save society money because they tend to die at a relatively young age, while nonsmokers tend to develop chronic diseases later in life and rack up huge medical bills (Barendregt, Bonneux, and van der Mass, 1997). Moreover, the SARS outbreak of 2003 did not create widespread economic panic in part because it disproportionately affects the elderly ("Epidemics and Economics," 2003). This then raises the question, If premature death is associated with a reduction in future medical costs, should these savings be included in a cost-effectiveness analysis?

The Panel on Cost-Effectiveness in Health and Medicine decided to put its theoretical concerns aside and allow researchers to exclude these future medical costs among survivors from the analysis. However, if future medical costs are likely to have a large impact on the analysis, the panel recommends that these costs be tested in a sensitivity analysis. This way, the analysis can be compared with studies that do not include such costs. Future medical costs are available using electronic data sources, such as MEPS.

CHAPTER

5

PROBABILITIES AND MODELS

OVERVIEW

IF COST-EFFECTIVENESS analysis were a building, probabilities would be its scaffolding. Probabilities indicate how likely subjects are to become ill, how likely subjects are to see a doctor, and so on. Therefore, they provide a framework for deciding how much an intervention will cost and how effective it will be.

A decision analysis model is essentially a series of values (such as costs or HRQL scores) bound together by a series of probabilities. In this chapter, you will get a general overview of probabilities and then begin the process of learning how they tie together to form a decision analysis model.

■ ■ ■

PROBABILITIES

So far, we've managed to get our research question in order and have created a basic chart outlining what we need to do in order to finish our analysis. We've also taken the first step toward understanding cost data, so we now have a rough understanding of how to work with the costs that go into each box in an event pathway. Now let's imagine that we've dug through the medical literature and datasets and found the probabilities and

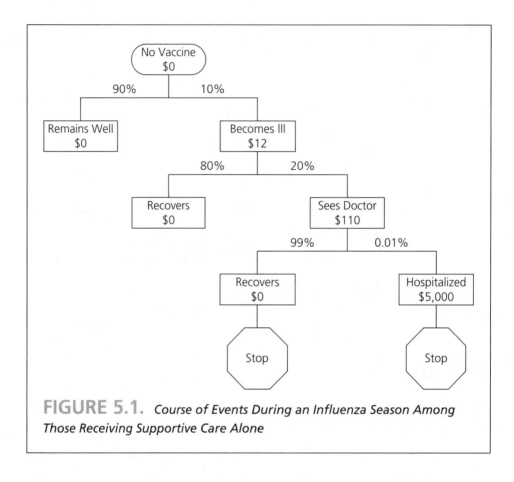

FIGURE 5.1. *Course of Events During an Influenza Season Among Those Receiving Supportive Care Alone*

costs needed to estimate the overall cost of each strategy. In this chapter, we'll see how to combine costs and probabilities and how to build a decision analysis model.

In Figure 5.1, we see a magnified view of the natural course of events for people who were not vaccinated at the start of influenza season. First, we need to know the chance that someone will become ill. Second, we need to know the probability that someone with the flu will stay at home rather than see a doctor. In Chapters Two and Four, we mentioned that *not* seeing a doctor can be associated with costs (because the patient ends up getting sick and hospitalized, or because the patient ends up infecting others) or savings (because the patient avoids the cost of the doctor's visit). For now, let's assume that staying at home does not cost or save any money.

In Figure 5.2, we see the vaccination side of the event pathway. The probabilities in this event pathway need to be specific to those who have received a vaccination. The vaccine not only alters the chance of becoming ill, but it also alters the chance of seeing a doctor or being hospitalized if you do become ill. (Recall that some people get a mild illness when exposed to the virus even though they were vaccinated.)

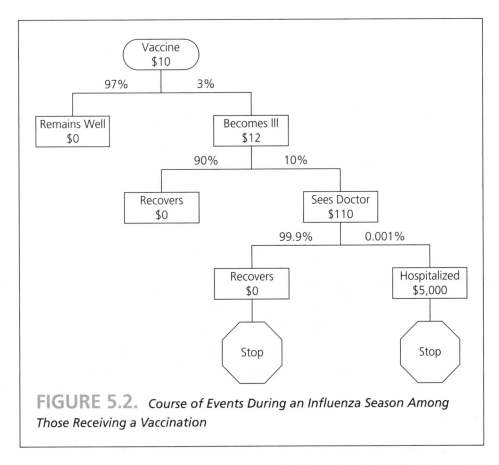

FIGURE 5.2. *Course of Events During an Influenza Season Among Those Receiving a Vaccination*

Now let's turn to costs. The cost of a doctor's visit or a hospitalization is not going to be much different among those who have or have not received a vaccination, and the cost of illness and hospitalization will be similar too. The main difference is that everyone in the vaccine arm gets a vaccination, and the probability of getting sick is lower. So in Figures 5.1 and 5.2, we see that we have to collect information on (1) the cost of the vaccine, (2) the cost of illness in general (for example, the cost of over-the-counter flu remedies), (3) the cost of the doctor's visit, and (4) the cost of hospitalization.

Glancing at Figures 5.1 and 5.2, it seems that vaccination is a no-brainer. There is a much lower chance of getting sick, seeing a doctor, and getting hospitalized among those who have been vaccinated. In fact, as we'll see in a minute, the total cost of illness among those who have received a vaccine is just $38, while those who have not will, on average, rack up a total cost of $84.

But one element is missing from these calculations: everyone in the vaccinate pathway will incur a $10 vaccine cost (top of Figure 5.2). If no one gets ill, then everyone in the vaccinate arm will still incur the $10 vaccine cost; if everyone gets a

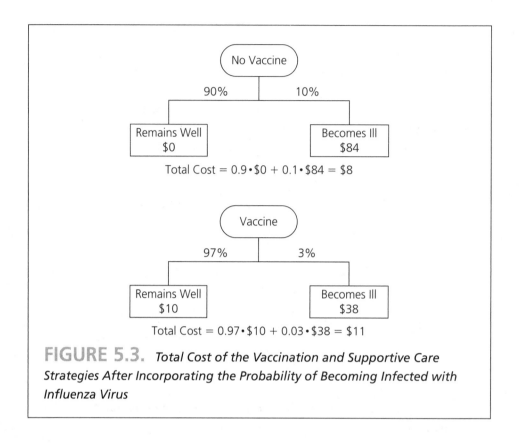

FIGURE 5.3.   *Total Cost of the Vaccination and Supportive Care Strategies After Incorporating the Probability of Becoming Infected with Influenza Virus*

vaccination at the beginning of the season but there was no outbreak of influenza, the money spent on vaccination would have been wasted. But if everyone is exposed to the virus, the group getting the vaccine is probably going to have lower total costs. Therefore, the chance of becoming ill (the incidence of the flu) becomes a critical determinant of the cost-effectiveness of vaccination. Let's see how adding the incidence of influenza virus infection changes things. (See Figure 5.3.)

For a moment, suspend disbelief and accept that the total cost of providing supportive care is $84 for each person who becomes ill with influenza. If there is a 10 percent chance of becoming infected, the average person in society will incur a cost of about $84 × 0.1 = $8.40. Among those who receive vaccination, everyone incurs the $10 cost, but the rate of symptomatic infection is 3 percent rather than 10 percent because these people were vaccinated. Of the 3 percent who become infected despite vaccination, total medical costs are lower. Why, you might ask, are the overall costs lower when the cost of a hospitalization or doctor's visit are similar? Remember that vaccinated people have a milder illness because they are partially protected. Thus, there is a lower chance of seeing a doctor or getting hospitalized even among those who do get ill.

Because the vaccine is only 70 effective at preventing the flu, 30 percent of all subjects in the influenza arm will become ill when exposed to the virus even though they were vaccinated. Thus, 30 percent of the 10 percent of those exposed to the flu virus (3 percent of all subjects) will become ill despite vaccination, and 97 percent will remain well. Therefore, in the vaccination arm, 97 percent incur only the $10 vaccine cost, and 3 percent incur the $38 cost of the flu ($28 for the medical care they receive while ill and $10 for the vaccine that failed to protect them). The average cost among vaccinated persons is thus $0.97 \times \$10 + 0.03 \times \$38 = \$10.84$, or about $11. Thus, if the incidence of influenza virus infection is 10 percent, the total cost of the vaccination strategy is $11 and the overall cost of the supportive care strategy is $8.

EXERCISE 1

1. What is the cost of the supportive care and vaccination strategies if the incidence rate of influenza virus infection is just 1 percent?

This is by no means the end of the story, of course. For one thing, we've neglected the effectiveness side of the equation. For another, we need to know what happens once we consider error in the cost and probability values we've entered into the event pathway. Finally, we want to include other relevant costs, such as the probability of secondary transmission. (See Figure 4.2.)

You now know about all there is to know about setting up a basic cost-effectiveness analysis. Doing the calculations by hand wasn't too difficult. However, the more elements you add to the event pathway, the trickier things get. Fortunately, there is a helpful shortcut to performing calculations within the event pathway sketches. This shortcut is called a decision analysis model.

PROJECT MAP

1. Think through your research question.
2. Sketch out the analysis.
3. Collect data for your model.
4. Adjust data.
5. *Build your model.*
6. Run and test the model.
7. Conduct sensitivity analysis.
8. Write it up.

DECISION ANALYSIS MODELS

An alternative way of representing an event pathway is with a **decision analysis model**. A decision analysis model calculates the costs and effects associated with events in an event pathway. Figure 5.4 is called a simple decision tree and is essentially the event pathway flipped on its side.

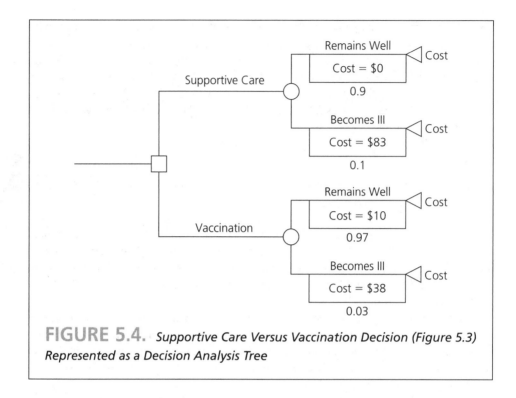

FIGURE 5.4. *Supportive Care Versus Vaccination Decision (Figure 5.3) Represented as a Decision Analysis Tree*

In this figure, both competing alternatives (vaccination and supportive care) are fused together, and this is represented as a square box. This box is called a *decision node*. The decision node is like a referee holding the competing alternatives apart as they set out to do battle. Following this square, you'll see a circle. The circle is called a *chance node*. A chance node is followed by two or more possible outcomes. In this case, the outcomes are Remains Well and Becomes Ill. The stop signs in Figures 5.1 and 5.2 are represented in a decision analysis model as a triangle at the very end of the model.

FOR EXAMPLE

Basic Components of a Decision Analysis Model

Basic decision analysis models have four components: (1) a decision node (usually represented as a square), (2) branches (lines), (3) chance nodes (circles), and (4) terminal nodes (triangles). The decision node indicates which choices we wish to evaluate, the chance node indicates the probabilities of two or more possible events, and the terminal node indicates the end points we wish to evaluate.

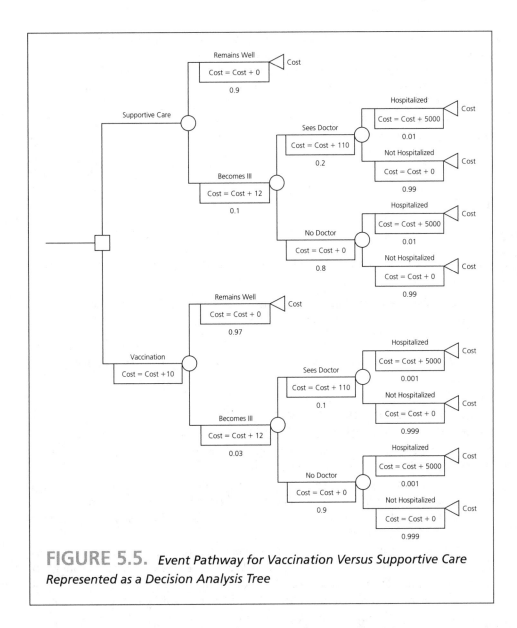

FIGURE 5.5. *Event Pathway for Vaccination Versus Supportive Care Represented as a Decision Analysis Tree*

Notice also in Figure 5.4 that, as in the event pathway, each box is represented as a cost. Also, each decision is associated with a probability. The probabilities in Figure 5.4 are located just below the cost.

As in Figure 5.3, we see that there is a $0.97 \times \$10 + 0.03 \times \$38 = \$11$ average cost among the vaccinated and a $0.1 \times \$84 + 0.9 \times \$0 = \$8$ average cost among those receiving supportive care alone.

Let's see what the decision analysis model looks like when the whole pathway is represented. In Figure 5.5, the incidence of influenza is 10 percent.

In Figure 5.5, the cost of each event is represented as a variable named Cost. The Cost variable is a running total of the costs of each event in a given event pathway. At each box in the tree, the running total is increased by the cost assigned to the box. For instance, everyone who receives a vaccination incurs a cost of $10 for the vaccine. For those who remain well, the total cost is $10 (for the vaccine) + $0 (remains well) = $10. For those who become ill despite vaccination, subjects also incur the initial cost of illness ($12 for aspirin and flu medications). If they do not see a doctor and are not hospitalized (the path along the bottom of Figure 5.5), the total cost is $10 (vaccine) + $12 (flu medications) + $0 (no doctor) + $0 (no hospitalization) = $22. Therefore, the final value of the variable Cost at the end of the bottom pathway in the figure is $22.

EXERCISES 2 TO 4

2. What is the total value of the Cost variable for a subject in the Supportive Care arm who sees a doctor and is subsequently hospitalized?

3. What is the total value of the Cost variable for subjects who do not see a doctor and are not subsequently hospitalized in the Supportive Care arm?

4. What is the *average* value of the variable Cost in the Sees Doctor branch of the Supportive Care arm? (Hint: Use the probability of incurring each cost to calculate the average value.)

Calculating the Cost of Each Strategy

Previously you were asked to take it on faith that the cost of supportive care for infected people is $84 and the cost of care for vaccinated persons who become ill anyway is $38. Now we'll see how to get these numbers.

Imagine that you were evaluating 100 subjects at the beginning of influenza season and that the flowchart in Figures 5.1 and 5.2 is a giant funnel. If you poured the subjects into the top of the flowchart, they would trickle through it, some going one way and others going the other way.

Subjects who trickle through a given box incur that cost. So a subject who becomes ill in the Supportive Care arm incurs a cost of $12 for over-the-counter medications. If he then sees a doctor, he adds $110 to this cost and has now collected a total cost of $122. If he then recovers, his total cost is $122. The probability of trickling into any given box is the probability of incurring that cost.

In Figure 5.6, the costs have been added up at the end of each terminal node. Working backward from each chance node, you'll see the total overall cost for that node. For instance, the total cost of the Sees Doctor node in the Supportive Care arm of the model is $5,122 × 0.01 + $122 × 0.99 = $172. The total cost of the No Doctor branch in the Supportive Care arm is $62 ($5,012 × 0.01 + $12 × 0.99 = $62). Now move one step back and look at the Becomes Ill branch. At this branch of the tree, the total cost is the average cost of the Sees Doctor branch and the No Doctor branches, or $172 × 0.2 + $62 × 0.8 = $84.

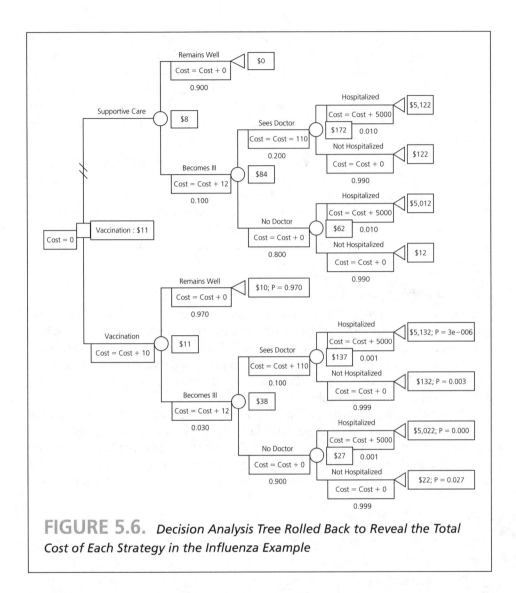

FIGURE 5.6. *Decision Analysis Tree Rolled Back to Reveal the Total Cost of Each Strategy in the Influenza Example*

The total cost of the Supportive Care arm of the study is the average of the Remains Well and the Becomes Ill costs, or $0.1 \times \$84 + 0.9 \times \$0 = \$8.40$ (or about $8). In other words, the total cost of the strategy is the weighted average cost of all branches emanating from that strategy.

TIPS AND TRICKS

At this point, you might be wondering why everything is rounded off to the nearest dollar. That's to get you used to rounding, which is the general rule in cost-effectiveness analysis. Cost-effectiveness researchers are a bit more honest than others in that they admit that the estimates are rough. In many scientific studies, you'll see estimates rounded to two decimal places. For instance, it's not uncommon to see a risk ratio of 1.22 or 3.54. Sure, that was the estimate for that group of people at that particular time in those particular circumstances. But if you do the study again, you'll probably not get a number that's even in the confidence interval of the original estimate. In cost-effectiveness analysis, it's not uncommon to give the reader a little wink and a nudge with a number like $12,000 per QALY gained when the number the researcher obtained is $12,431 per QALY gained.

Thus, if we believe the figures we've entered so far, the overall cost of the vaccination strategy ($11) is about $3 higher than the cost of the supportive care strategy ($8), which is exactly what we found in the previous section when we calculated the values by hand. In the next few chapters, we'll see what happens when we test these values and add effectiveness information. Before going there, though, let's place what you have already learned about decision analysis models into perspective.

The Idea Behind Decision Analysis

Imagine that you have $100,000 to invest. You've always wanted to study public health, but you've also dreamed about writing a novel. If you write a novel, you reason, you can simply invest the money in a mutual fund and earn interest, making small withdrawals as needed. Since you are undecided between the two options, you examine which will be the better option financially. Decision analysis is a tool for making decisions using statistical probabilities.

Decision analysis is based on a concept called **expected value**, in which the value of an uncertain event (such as making $10,000 in the stock market) is weighed against the chances that the event will occur. For example, if you know that the historical average increase in a particular mutual fund is 10 percent per year, then the expected value of the return on your $100,000 investment is $0.1 \times \$100,000 = \$10,000$ over one year.

TIPS AND TRICKS

For the expected value calculations to be correct, all probabilities in a decision tree must be independent (mutually exclusive).

The expected value also refers to the weighted average value of all costs or effectiveness outcomes in a decision analysis tree. In Figure 5.6, for instance, the expected value of vaccination was $11, and the expected value of supportive care was $8. If we were trying to spend less money, we would choose supportive care based on the limited information presented by that model. However, if we were trying to make a decision based on how to maximize income (as in the book versus public health school example), we would choose the decision with the highest expected value.

Let's return to that example. You set your sights five years down the road and assume that if you go to public health school, all of the $100,000 would be spent on your education after living expenses are taken into account, but you would be able to earn about $50,000 per year working in public health after graduation. After taxes and living expenses, you estimate that you would save about $10,000 over the three years after graduation.

If you decide to write a novel, you will have spent your $100,000, along with the interest on the mutual fund, on living expenses over the five-year period. If you publish the novel, you could earn an additional $30,000. Your college English professor advises you that there is about a 1 percent chance that you will be published. Therefore, the "invest and write" option will produce a return of $30,000 $\times$ 0.01 = $300.00.

Since $10,000 is more than $300, you might go for the career in public health. However, you might not be satisfied with your calculations; there is a chance that the mutual fund could do very well, but there is also a chance that you could lose money. If it does well, you could end up with leftover money from your mutual fund investment at the end of five years. So if you write the book, you might make money even if you don't publish. But if the mutual fund loses money, you might not be able to finish your novel, which would be quite depressing.

There is also a chance that you will not find a job right out of public health school. Using a decision analysis model, you can estimate the ranges of possible earnings associated with each decision at the end of the five-year period. Ideally, you would want a rough idea not only of the average earnings associated with each decision, but also the chance that you will end up in the gutter with a bottle of wine if you choose one over the other. This way, you'll not only have a better idea of which decision is riskier but you'll also know the chances of a very bad outcome.

FOR EXAMPLE

Why You'll Never Catch a Decision Analyst in a Casino

Gambling casinos, like decision analysis models, use the concept of expected value to ensure that they will profit off gamblers. For the casino to profit, earnings at tables and slot machines must, on average, be greater than the casino's expenses. Casinos tend to employ a large staff and have spectacular displays of opulence, such as re-creations of downtown Manhattan in miniature. Thus, the probability that the client will lose must be significantly greater than the probability of winning if the casino wishes to keep its doors open. Although the occasional winner will surface from a wild night of gambling, the average person can expect to lose money.

Recall that technical types call the various options that you are deciding between *competing alternatives*. Decision analysis can thus be described as the process of making an optimal choice among competing alternatives under conditions of uncertainty. In the case of cost-effectiveness analysis, the competing alternatives are the different medical interventions we are studying.

In the past, researchers performing a cost-effectiveness analysis had to write a computer program that would calculate the cost and effectiveness of different medical interventions, or attempt to calculate all of the costs and probabilities on a spreadsheet. Today most cost-effectiveness analyses can be easily assembled using decision analysis software.

You have already learned the basics of building a decision analysis model. The basic functions of all decision analysis software packages are more or less similar. If you choose to follow the examples provided here using decision analysis software, you will get a better understanding of the concepts behind decision analysis. Tips on using different software packages are also provided throughout this book. A list of software packages with online links and evaluations is provided at http://www.pceo.org. Many of these companies offer free trial versions of their software.

Types of Decision Analysis Models

There are a number of types of decision analysis models. The most basic is a **simple decision analysis tree** model. Simple decision trees are usually employed to examine events that will occur in the near future. They are therefore best suited to evaluate interventions to prevent or treat illnesses of a short duration, such as acute infectious diseases. They may also be used to evaluate chronic diseases that may be cured (for example, by surgical intervention). When these trees are used to evaluate diseases that change over time, they sometimes become too unruly to be useful.

For chronic or complex diseases, it is best to use a **state transition model**. This type of model allows researchers to incorporate changes in health states over time into the analysis. For example, if a person has cancer, there is a chance that the person will recover within a year and then relapse. There is also a chance that the person will remain sick for some time or will die soon. With every passing month (or year), the chances of survival, recovery, or deterioration change. These models, which are also called **Markov models**, allow researchers to track changes in the quality of life, the quantity of life, and the cost of a disease over time when different health interventions are applied.

In the next chapter, we'll put Markov models to the test, and use them to estimate changes in life expectancy associated with a given intervention.

CHAPTER

6

CALCULATING LIFE EXPECTANCY

OVERVIEW

SO FAR, you've learned how to work with costs and how to enter them into a decision analysis model. You now know that the probabilistically weighted cost of each competing alternative is called the expected value of that strategy. Costs, though, are just one component of the expected value. The expected value of QALYs—the quality and quantity of life among people receiving each strategy—is the most important component of a cost-effectiveness analysis.

In this chapter, we first take a quick look at how to calculate changes in years gained when an intervention is administered using a hand calculator or spreadsheet program. Then we see how this is done using a Markov model. In the next chapter, you will learn about health-related quality-of-life (also known by the acronym HRQL) scores. You will learn how to adjust life expectancy for health-related quality of life to calculate QALYs in Chapter Eight.

■ ■ ■

HAND-CALCULATING YEARS GAINED

If we are studying vaccination against the influenza virus, we'll first want to know how many deaths would have occurred without vaccination. These data can be obtained from death certificate records, prospective studies, or national health surveys that have been linked to mortality data. (Data sources are covered in detail in Chapter Twelve.) In this example, we'll use hypothetical data to simplify things a bit.

Suppose our hypothetical cohort consists of healthy people aged 15 to 65. Our research question might assume the form: "Is vaccination more cost-effective than supportive care among healthy people aged 15 to 65 in the United States?" We'll define the supportive care as, "Do not vaccinate people, and treat the flu symptoms if they become ill." Let's say that we are evaluating a work- and school-based vaccination strategy, in which just about everyone has to get vaccinated.

FOR EXAMPLE

Whom Are We Studying?

One perpetual problem in cost-effectiveness analysis is matching the demographic characteristics of the cohort in the datasets or research papers you are using to the demographic characteristics of the cohort in your research question. If we found an article on influenza-related deaths that used older wealthy white people as subjects, the mortality rate might be very different from the rate we wish to use in a study looking at a younger representative sample of the U.S. population.

One way to conduct the analysis is to look at the age at which unvaccinated people died of influenza (Table 6.1). If we knew their average life expectancy at the age that each subject actually died, we could then add all of the life years lost across all subjects. For instance, if the average twenty-year-old has a life expectancy of 78.5 years, then an influenza death at age twenty results in the total loss of 78.5 years − 20 years = 58.5 years.

The remaining life expectancy for people of any given age can be obtained from a life table. U.S. life tables are available from the National Center for Health Statistics (http://www.cdc.gov/nchs). Links to life tables from other countries can be found using a search engine. The Organization for Economic Cooperation and Development is a good source for developed countries and the World Health Organization for industrializing nations.

Life tables for the United States in 2003 are provided in Appendix B. Check out this appendix now so that you can see where I am getting our data from. In the appendix, the final column of the first table contains the information we are looking

TABLE 6.1. **Number of Deaths Due to Influenza Virus Infection, by Age Group**

Age	Annual Number of Deaths
15 to 24 years	6
25 to 34 years	11
35 to 44 years	24
45 to 54 years	54
55 to 64 years	69

for: the remaining life expectancy for each age group. Most life tables you encounter will be similar. Appendix B also has life expectancy at a given age by race and gender in the United States.

Table 6.2 contains deaths, the mean age of death due to the flu, and life expectancy (had the subject survived the influenza infection) by age group for our hypothetical

TABLE 6.2. **Deaths, Mean Age of Death Due to Influenza Virus Infection, and Life Expectancy for Persons Aged 15 to 65**

Age	Deaths Due to Influenza (1)	Midpoint Age in Interval (2)	Life Expectancy at Midpoint (3)
15 to 24 years	6	20	78.5
25 to 34 years	11	30	79
35 to 44 years	24	40	79.6
45 to 54 years	54	50	80.6
55 to 64 years	69	60	82.3

FOR EXAMPLE

Growing Older, Living Longer

Some students may wonder why they need a life table to figure out the mean age of death for people from a given age group if you already know what human life expectancy is. After all, if life expectancy is 78 years in your country and a person dies at age 40, one could just assume that he lost 78 − 40 = 38 years of life. The bad news is that people in different age groups have ever expanding life expectancies, so you always have to look up the life expectancy at any given age. The good news is that *your* life expectancy is longer than you might think. (So you are wasting fewer precious moments of life reading this book than you first imagined.)

As it turns out, human life expectancy at birth in the United States is somewhere around 78 years. But as we grow older, our life expectancy grows with us. For instance, 70 year olds can expect to live a full additional fifteen years to age 85. The reason is that those who make it past birth trauma have gotten a good deal of risk behind them. Those with serious illness or risk factors for premature mortality such as smoking tend to die younger too. Thus, the healthiest people make it to age 70, and, because they are healthier, they have more life to look forward to. The other bit of good news is that life expectancy at birth also tends to increase from one year to the next in most countries, thanks in part to the appropriate use of health interventions. In fact, life expectancy for males in the United States was just 48 years at the turn of the twentieth century (National Center for Health Statistics, 2005).

cohort of 15 to 65 year olds. One important part of this table is the midpoint of each age interval. Assuming that someone who is 15 years old is just about as likely to die as someone who is 25, the average age of death among 15 to 25 year olds will be about (15 years of age + 25 years of age)/2 = 20 years of age. (In Table 6.2, the 15-to-24 age interval represents everyone who just turned 15 to everyone who is 24 years and 364 days and 23 hours old, so the midpoint is 20 years.)

In the influenza study, we are interested only in subjects aged 15 to 65. Nonetheless, someone who dies at age 64 still loses around 20 years of life. Therefore, a death even at this age counts for a lot of lost life expectancy.

From the information in Table 6.2, we can easily calculate the total years of life lost to influenza infection in the cohort (see Table 6.3). This is just equal to the life expectancy at that age (column 3 of Table 6.3) minus the mean age of death due to influenza virus infection (column 2). The total years of life lost among all people in

TABLE 6.3. **Calculating Total Years of Life Lost Due to Influenza Virus Infection in the United States**

Age	Deaths Due to Influenza (1)	Midpoint Age (2)	Life Expectancy at Age (From Life Table) (3)	Years of Life Lost per Person (Col. 3 − Col. 4) (4)	Total Years of Life Lost (Col. 1 × Col. 4) (5)
15 to 24 years	6	20	78.5	58.5	351
25 to 34 years	11	30	79	49	539
35 to 44 years	24	40	79.6	39.6	950
45 to 54 years	54	50	80.6	30.6	1,652
55 to 64 years	69	60	82.3	22.3	1,539
Total	164				5,032

each age interval is the number of deaths (column 1) times the average number of years of life lost per person (column 4).

To obtain the total years of life lost due to influenza virus infections, add across the age groups. At the bottom of Table 6.3, we thus see that just over 5,000 years of life are lost annually in the United States due to influenza virus infection among otherwise healthy 15 to 65 year olds. This is the total quantity of life we would expect to lose in the supportive care arm of our analysis.

So how many additional life years would we get from vaccination? In the research question posed above, we are evaluating a scenario in which nearly everyone gets vaccinated. One estimate is that because the efficacy of the vaccine is 70 percent, we could prevent 70 percent of all deaths, and therefore 70 percent of all years of life that would otherwise have been lost. Thus, we might estimate that we can prevent 5,000 years of life × 0.7 = 3,500 years of life that would otherwise have been lost.

However, some students of public health may be familiar with the concept of *herd immunity*. Herd immunity occurs when the level of vaccination is so high that the virus fizzles out altogether, and no cases of disease remain. If we believe that we can achieve herd immunity, we would prevent all 5,000 years of life lost. (This is one example of the difference between efficacy and effectiveness.)

Stop here for a moment and think about the implications of this. This is $164 \times 0.7 = 115$ lives saved. Among those people, there are about 3,500 total extra years of life enjoyed by these 115 people. These are mothers, fathers, children, and spouses who would still be alive at the end of the influenza season if the government followed your recommendations to provide vaccination to everyone in the United States (that is, in this hypothetical example). But if you found that vaccination were costly relative to other things done in health, you could be saving more lives by directing needed resources to more important lifesaving interventions.

FOR EXAMPLE

How to Save Lives Through Inaction

You learned earlier in the book that if you have a fixed amount of funding for health care, cost-effectiveness analysis will tell you how to maximize the total number of lives you are saving with those scarce resources. But what if you don't have a fixed amount to spend, such as occurs in private sector health systems? In the United States, clinicians often order loads of medical tests when the patient comes to see them, many of which are known to be cost-ineffective. There is also a tendency to use the newest and most expensive therapies. All of this is justified on the grounds that it just might save a life. After all, a clinician might reason, what is money relative to precious life? In reality, all of this unnecessary care probably raises insurance premiums. This increased cost forces many employers to drop insurance carriers. It also pushes those who pay for insurance on their own out of the insurance market. Given that insurance itself is probably lifesaving and is a fairly efficient medical expenditure (Muennig and others, 2005), forcing people out of the insurance market can increase overall mortality. Therefore, clinicians who mistakenly believe that they are helping their patients with excessive testing and treatment may in fact be killing unseen people.

CALCULATING LIFE YEARS LOST USING MARKOV MODELS

Let's take a look at how our influenza analysis might progress had we used year-to-year data rather than age intervals. Suppose that instead of the deaths in Table 6.3, we followed a cohort of 1 million unvaccinated 15 year olds between the ages of 15 and 100. (This requires a leap of faith, but stick with me here.)

Any one of these 1 million folks can survive to the next age, die of influenza, or die of something else. In Table 6.4, column 2 represents deaths due to influenza,

TABLE 6.4. **Total Deaths, Deaths Due to Influenza Virus Infection, and Total Survivors in a Cohort of 1 Million 15 Year Olds**

Age	Deaths Due to Any Cause (1)	Died from Influenza (2)	Total Surviving (3)
15	407	1	1,000,000
16	575	0	999,593
17	683	0	999,018
18	728	2	998,335
19	734	0	997,607
20	898	0	996,873
. . .	. . .	. . .	. . .
95	11,589	0	29,011
96	8,754	0	17,422
97	3,989	0	8,668
98	1,234	0	4,679
99	2,038	0	3,445
100	664	0	1,407

column 1 represents deaths due to all causes, and column 3 the total number of people surviving each year of life. (Note that there are no deaths due to influenza virus infection recorded after the age of 65 because we are interested only in deaths due to influenza among people between the ages of 15 and 65.) Table 6.4 has been truncated so that it fits in the book.

TIPS AND TRICKS

Over one hundred years of education research, dating back to the great John Dewey, has shown that students learn best by doing. From this point on, I highly recommend that students with access to a computer follow along on a spreadsheet using the examples in the book. You will find full tables and free spreadsheet software at http://www.pceo.org/learn.html.

In Table 6.4, we start with 1 million 15 year olds (column 3), but 407 die in the first year (column 1). This leaves $1,000,000 - 407 = 999,593$ survivors at age 16.

Suppose that we wish to calculate the total number of years lived by this cohort of 1 million 15 year olds. You might be thinking that this is just the sum total of column 3 values in Table 6.4. After all, each interval is one year in length and those are the total number of people alive each year. That's true, but remember that people who die don't all die on January 1. On average, the 407 15 year olds dying in row 1, column 1 of Table 6.4 will die about six months into the year (in June). All those dying will therefore have lived about half a year on average, and we need to count this additional life. Because the 407 people who died between the ages of 15 and 16 lived a half-year of life on average, we subtract $407/2 = 203.5$ rather than all 407 years of life for that year.

TIPS AND TRICKS

To generate Table 6.5 using the electronic version of Table 6.4, simply add a column after the Total Surviving column; name it "Person-Years," and perform the calculations. To enter the formula, type "$= D2 - B2 * 0.5$" (without the quotes). Next, click on the cell in which you just entered the formula (cell E2). The cell will appear highlighted. Grab the lower right-hand side of the cell. It should turn into a plus sign. Now drag it all the way down to the final age group. The spreadsheet program should have done all of the calculations for you, so that you don't have to reenter the formula in each cell. If it doesn't work on the first try, try again. You'll get the hang of it eventually.

As shown in Table 6.5, this half-year correction is calculated as column 1 − column 2 × 0.5. The number of years of life lived by a group of people is referred to as *person-years*. Thus, there were 997,797 person-years lived between the ages of 15 and 16. If we sum all person-years together, we find that this cohort lived 63,670,217 person-years between the ages of 15 and 100.

We can also calculate the number of years lived by the average person in the cohort. To obtain this average, we would simply divide the total number of years lived (person-years) between the ages 15 and 100 by the total number of people at the start of the study. The average number of years lived by the average 15 year old is also known as the life expectancy at age 15. In this case, it would be 63,670,217 person-years/1,000,000 persons = 63.67 years. This is precisely how life expectancy was calculated in the life table in Appendix B by the grownups at the National Center for Health Statistics.

Now we have the total person-years and life expectancy of people in this cohort of 1 million unvaccinated 15 year olds (regardless of whether they died of the flu). How do we get the incremental gain in person-years or life expectancy among those who have received the influenza vaccination? To make things simple, let's say that the

TABLE 6.5. **Total Person-Years Lived by the Cohort of 1 Million 15 Year Olds**

Age	Alive (1)	All Deaths (2)	Person-Years (Col. 1 − Col. 2 × 0.5) (3)
15	1,000,000	407	999,797
16	999,593	575	999,306
17	999,018	683	998,677
18	998,335	728	997,971
19	997,607	734	997,240
20	996,873	898	996,424
. . .	. . .	. . .	. . .
95	29,011	11,589	23,217
96	17,422	8,754	13,045
97	8,668	3,989	6,674
98	4,679	1,234	4,062
99	3,445	2,038	2,426
100	1,407	664	1,075
Total	64,169,845		63,670,217

influenza vaccine is 100 percent effective. Now we repeat this process with and without the deaths due to influenza virus infection (see Table 6.6).

As you can see from Table 6.6, the gain in person years is 63,670,217 − 63,678,453 = 8,236 person-years. Note that we stopped exposing the subjects to influenza once they hit age 65. Thus, the total number of deaths in the age groups 95 through 100 is identical. However, there are fewer survivors going forward in the unvaccinated group.

TABLE 6.6. Person-Years Lived Among the Cohort of 15 Year Olds, Including and Excluding Deaths Due to Influenza Virus Infection

	All Deaths			All Deaths But Influenza-Related Deaths		
Age	All Deaths (Unvaccinated)	Total Surviving	Person-Years	Total Deaths Less Influenza Deaths	Total Surviving	Person-Years Less Influenza
15	407	1,000,000	999,797	406	1,000,000	999,797
16	575	999,593	999,306	575	999,594	999,307
17	683	999,018	998,677	683	999,019	998,678
18	728	998,335	997,971	726	998,336	997,973
19	734	997,607	997,240	734	997,610	997,243
20	898	996,873	996,424	898	996,876	996,427
. . .	. . .	. . .	. . .	. . .	. . .	. . .
95	11,589	29,011	23,217	11,589	29,175	23,381
96	8,754	17,422	13,045	8,754	17,586	13,209
97	3,989	8,668	6,674	3,989	8,832	6,838
98	1,234	4,679	4,062	1,234	4,843	4,226
99	2,038	3,445	2,426	2,038	3,609	2,590
100	664	1,407	1,075	664	1,571	1,239
Total			63,670,217			63,678,453

TIPS AND TRICKS

If we divide the number of deaths by the number of survivors in Table 6.6, we obtain the **mortality rate**. The mortality rate at any given age in this example is equal to the probability of death at that age. Most often we will know the mortality rate in the cohort, but not the total number of deaths. So how do we recreate it? The number of deaths at any age is equal to the product of the total number of survivors at any given age and the mortality rate for persons of that age or in that age group (see Table 6.7).

TABLE 6.7. **Age-Specific Mortality Rates, Survivors, and Number of Deaths in the Cohort of 1 Million 15-Year-Old Subjects**

Age	Mortality Rate (1)	Alive (2)	All Deaths (Col. 1 × Col. 2) (3)
15	0.0004	1,000,000	407
16	0.0006	999,593	575
17	0.0007	999,018	683
18	0.0007	998,335	728
19	0.0007	997,607	734
20	0.0009	996,873	898
. . .	. . .	. . .	. . .
95	0.3995	29,011	11,589
96	0.5025	17,422	8,754
97	0.4602	8,668	3,989
98	0.2637	4,679	1,234
99	0.5915	3,445	2,038
100	0.4718	1,407	664

It may not be a surprise to most of you that this whole process can be modeled in a way that is quick and versatile. What will be surprising is how easy it is to become a supermodeler using standard software.

Principles of Markov Modeling

Most interventions have some component of time to them. For instance, to model screening mammography, we must have some way to measure the way that breast cancer progresses over time when left untreated. We must also account for changes over time among women who are treated for the disease but not cured. Moreover, we don't provide screening mammography just once. We might provide it every six months or once every five years.

To model events that unfold over time, we want some sort of **recursive** component in our model. A recursive event is one that repeats over and over. For example, if we were evaluating screening for high blood pressure, we might want to capture the cost of diagnosing and treating high blood pressure in year 1 and then include the cost of ongoing treatment in years 2, 3, 4, and so on until the patient dies. (We never cure high blood pressure; we just provide symptomatic treatment.)

Recall from Chapter Five that a model that contains some component of time in it is called a state transition model or Markov model (Figure 6.1). Figure 6.1 can be thought of as a machine for shuffling people through time. The bent fork in the road represents the chance that any given subject will die in a particular year. Subjects are cycled through once per year. With each passing year, the number of subjects in the dead fork increases. The rate at which the number of subjects collect at the dead node is equal to the age-specific mortality rate.

Now you will see why we took you through the whole exercise of calculating person-years.

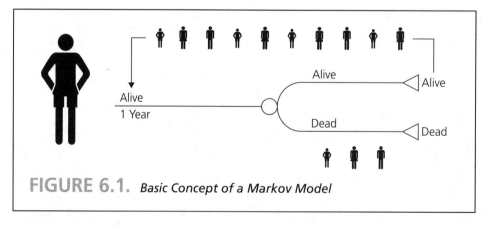

FIGURE 6.1. *Basic Concept of a Markov Model*

Note: Subjects start at time zero (the large figure). They are then exposed to a chance of death. Survivors gain one year and return to the start of the model, where they are again exposed to a chance of death. Those who die exit the model. This process is repeated until all subjects die. The mean number of times a subject passes through the model is equal to the life expectancy of the cohort.

NOTE

I have opted to describe Markov models in a way that is easy to understand. The actual way that the computer performs these calculations differs somewhat from what I describe here.

Subjects who are alive at the end of the first cycle of the model are assigned one person-year, and those who die are assigned no person years. Suppose that subjects die at the same age-specific mortality rate that they did in Table 6.5. If we start at age 15 and send 1 million subjects through eighty-five cycles to age 100, there will be 63,670,217 total person-years gained, and the average subject will have accrued 63.67 years. Said another way, *the average number of times survivors rotate through the model is equal to the average number of person-years lived by that cohort.* The average number of rotations is therefore equal to the life expectancy of the cohort.

TIPS AND TRICKS

You would be well served to take the time now to build your own Markov model. The online component of this book, the Program in Cost-Effectiveness and Outcomes, contains a downloadable laboratory manual with links to demo software and step-by-step exercises for building your own Markov models. See http://www.pceo.org/learn.html.

Using a Markov model, we can count more than the years that accrue as the model completes cycles. We can also count medical costs, living costs, health-related quality of life scores, or whatever else might be relevant for our analysis. For instance, suppose we are interested in calculating the lifelong cost associated with breast cancer in patients who have been diagnosed using a screening mammogram. We would start the model using the average age of onset of breast cancer. The number of survivors would be determined using the probability of death specific to women who have been diagnosed with breast cancer using screening mammography. Each patient who is still living at the end of the year gains one year of additional life (one person-year). But she can also be assigned medical costs, home health care costs, transportation costs, and so forth. Women who die do not accrue such costs, so these women neither gain a year of life nor accrue costs.

Thus, if the average annual cost of living with breast cancer were $10,000, a group of 10 women would incur a cost of 10 × $10,000 = $100,000 in year 1. Now imagine that by year 2, one woman died. Year 2 costs would then be 9 × $10,000 = $90,000. If we continued this process until the last subject died, we would not only have the average number of life years lived, but the total cost incurred by these women over that time period. (See Table 6.8.)

Markov Models in Practice

Let's take a moment to see how a Markov model works using DATA, a program produced by TreeAge Software (Figure 6.2). For a moment, we'll return to the influenza example so that you can see how Markov modeling works in its most basic form.

TABLE 6.8. **Progression of a Cohort of Ten Women with Breast Cancer over a Six-Year Period**

Year	Women Surviving	Discounted Years Lived[a]	Cost of Treating Breast Cancer[b]	Discounted Cost[a]
1	10	9.7	$100,000	$97,087
2	9	9.0	$90,000	$84,834
3	8	7.8	$80,000	$73,211
4	7	6.7	$70,000	$62,194
5	6	5.6	$60,000	$51,757
6	5	4.6	$50,000	$41,874
Total		**43**	**$450,000**	**$410,957**

[a]Beginning in January of the reference year at a 3 percent rate of discount.
[b]Costs in this column have not been half-year corrected for simplicity of presentation. In an actual analysis, it would be important to base the figures on person-years rather than the number of deaths.

The first thing that you come across in Figure 6.2 is a box that says "Markov Information" followed by "Term: _stage > 103." The "Term" in this case stands for "Termination," and tells the program how many one-year loops it is going to make before it stops. In this case, it will loop 103 times (or until all of the subjects are dead). The odd notation "_stage" is a function used by DATA to keep track of how many cycles have been completed. In this model, one cycle is one year; thus, when _stage is equal to 10, ten years have passed.

In this figure there is an initial Alive/Dead branch followed by another Alive/Dead branch. The first Alive/Dead branch (top) also contains a box called "Markov Information." This is followed by various reward ("Rwd") terms. For now, just consider the "Incr Rwd." This stands for incremental reward and tells the program what to add up every time a subject passes through the Alive branch. The incremental reward can be anything. For instance, it can be an annual medical bill for someone with breast cancer.

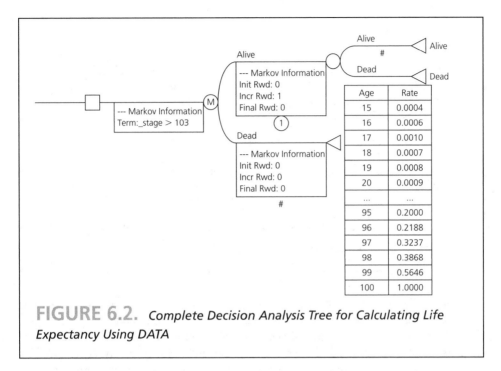

FIGURE 6.2. *Complete Decision Analysis Tree for Calculating Life Expectancy Using DATA*

The number sign (#) indicates 1−p. Thus, if the probability is 0.0004, the number sign assumes the value of 1 − 0.0004 = 0.9996.

For now let's count the incremental reward in years. In this figure, the incremental reward is set to 1 for the Alive branch and 0 for the Dead branch. Thus, every time a subject passes through the Alive branch, the running total reward is increased by one, representing one year of life. Every subject who dies gets a reward of zero (no additional years of life) and exits the model. (If this is all terribly depressing to you, just remember that these are hypothetical subjects.)

Note that below the "Markov Information" box on the Alive branch, you'll also find the number 1 (circled in Figure 6.2). This number indicates that at time zero (before the first loop), there is a 100 percent chance of being alive and moving forward into the model. This is followed by a circle (a chance node) and another Alive/Dead option. At this point, there is a chance of dying. In this figure, the chance of dying at any age is presented as a table.

For instance, following the previous example, it tells the program that when the subject is 15 years old, he has a 0.0004 chance of dying. To reiterate, there are two Alive/Dead branches, but only the second determines who lives and who dies. The first branch is used to either absorb the subjects who die or pass the subjects who survive back into the tree. For this reason, the first dead node is called the *absorbing state*.

Let's call the table in Figure 6.2 "tDead2003[age]." This reflects the age-specific probability of death in the United States in 2003. Again, every time a subject passes

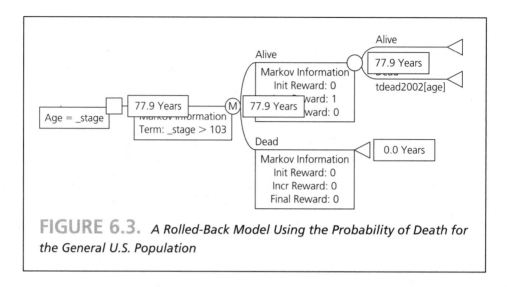

FIGURE 6.3. *A Rolled-Back Model Using the Probability of Death for the General U.S. Population*

through the Dead branch, no points are given, and the subject exits the model. Thus, when subjects are 20 years old, 0.0009 will die and accrue no points, but $1 - 0.0009 = 0.9991$ will live and accrue a reward equal to one year of life. When subjects are 95 years old, 0.2 (20 percent) will die, and 0.8 will live to see age 96.

If there is no chance of death (the values in tDead2003 are all equal to zero), the incremental reward will be 103 because we have told the model to stop cycling after 103 turns. Other things can cause the model to stop cycling as well. Most important, the model will stop looping once the total proportion of subjects remaining alive reaches zero.

Once the model stops looping, it presents the mean value of the incremental reward. In the previous section, you learned that if you add up the total number of survivors in a cohort, you end up with the total person-years in that cohort. You also learned that if you divide the sum of all person-years across age groups by the total number of people at the start of the cohort, you end up with the cohort's life expectancy. This is the expected value of the number of years lived by the average person in the cohort.

This expected value is obtained by **rolling back** the model. Figure 6.3 is the rolled-back version of a Markov model that uses the age-specific probability of death for the general population. The 77.9 years is the life expectancy of the cohort, and "P = 1" following the expected value indicates that the probability of achieving this value is 1.0. At the Dead branch, you'll see "0.0 Years; FP = 1." "FP" stands for "Final Proportion" and indicates that all subjects have died. The "0.0 Years" notation indicates that the sum of incremental reward values for all subjects who have passed through this branch is zero.

In the Alive branch, the final proportion of subjects in this branch of the tree is 0, and the total incremental value is 77.9 years.

TIPS AND TRICKS

Recall that all future values, whether costs or years of life, must be discounted at a rate of 3 percent. Fortunately, DATA has a function built in that allows all values to be discounted at a specified rate. The laboratory manual walks students through the process of entering the discounting function into DATA. In short, any value entered in the "Incremental" box must be discounted.

Soon, we will see how to assign costs (for example, cost of hospitalization, cost of a medical visit) to each year a subject survives. We'll also see how to enter health-related quality-of-life (HRQL) scores to calculate QALYs. First, though, we'll take a break from modeling and look at HRQL measures in more detail.

CHAPTER

7

WORKING WITH HEALTH-RELATED QUALITY-OF-LIFE MEASURES

OVERVIEW

RECALL THAT a quality-adjusted life year (QALY) may be thought of as a year of life that is lived in perfect health. In Chapter Two, we learned that HRQL scores assume a value between 0 and 1. This ratio may be simply thought of as a continuum of values ranging from perfect health to death. Thus, if a medical intervention adds 10 years of life and each of these years is associated with an HRQL of 0.7, the medical intervention would have resulted in a gain of 0.7 × 10 years = 7 years of perfect health (7 QALYs).

In this chapter, we take the first step toward calculating QALYs as we learn the basic theory behind HRQL scores, learn how to obtain HRQL scores for cost-effectiveness analyses, and learn how to use HRQL scores using worked examples.

NOTE

This section is implemented with a crescendo-like teaching technique in which information is broken into small parts and then reassembled into a workable whole. This may seem somewhat repetitive to some students, but it forces most people to learn the material more naturally and effectively.

FRAMEWORK

In this section, we briefly discuss the formal methods used to translate a person's perception of the quality of life in various health states into an HRQL score. It provides some definitions, a basic outline of how HRQL scores are generated, and finally a more detailed description of how these scores are collected and used. This will allow you to follow along with a clear understanding of how this process works. Keep in mind that these measures were designed with consistency, rather than specificity, as a primary objective (Gold, Franks, McCoy, and Fryback, 1998).

First, the definitions.

A **preference score** is a number between 0 and 1. Zero represents "I'd just as soon be dead," and one represents perfect health. For instance, a preference score of 0.7 represents 70 percent of the way between "I'd just as soon be dead" and "I'm in perfect health." Take this on faith for a moment.

Recall from Chapter One that health state reflects how well or how badly people are doing with respect to a given aspect of a particular disease or condition. For instance, not being able to get out of bed is a health state. So are moderate depression and having some pain. One's health status is the collection of health states.

Whereas a preference score refers to a single health state, an HRQL score is essentially an overall preference score for multiple health states. (Some experts will quibble with this, but it's confusing to think of an HRQL score in any other way.)

Second, this essentially is how HRQL scores are generated:

1. Preference scores for a set number of health states are obtained from a large sample of people. For instance, people will be asked to assign a preference score to "some mobility limitations" or "in severe pain."

2. Statistical analyses are conducted on these preference scores such that we know what a given health state is worth to the average person in the sample. For instance, we'll know that "some mobility limitations" has a preference score of 0.7.

3. These values are translated into a type of score sheet that requires the user to check off broad categories of health states. For instance, the score sheet might contain a category called "Mobility." The user is then required to check off one of three states: "No problems getting around," "Some problems getting around,"

and "Immobilized." It might also contain a category called pain that contains "no pain," "moderate pain," and "severe pain."

4. It translates these health states into an overall HRQL score. If the user checks "Some problems getting around" and "severe pain," the score sheet provides an overall HRQL score of, say, 0.3.

Now we'll examine these steps in detail. Obviously the steps just given provide a very basic outline. Immediate questions should pop into mind such as, "How does this translation happen?" Now all your questions will be answered.

Preference Scores

Preference scores are taken from a sample of subjects from the general population that is subjected to a series of exercises based on expected utility theory. Expected utility theory is little more than a way of turning health states such as level of pain into a number (the preference score).

The "utility" part of expected utility theory is the preference score for a given health state (for example, being unable to walk) when a person is otherwise in perfect health. For instance, given that the utility of perfect health is 1 and the utility of death is 0, a fellow in perfect health who cannot walk because of a war injury might have a preference score of 0.6. This indicates that to the average person who cannot walk but is in otherwise perfect health, each moment of life is worth 60 percent of that of a person who can fully walk.

The "expected" part of "expected utility theory" implies that these utilities are derived by calculating expected values, as you would with a decision analysis model. How might such a decision analysis model look? Consider the **standard gamble** technique.

Suppose you had an illness that required you to remain in bed for the rest of your life, and an evil magician appeared at your bedside. This magician told you that you could either remain as you are for the rest of your life or play a potentially deadly game. If you won this game, you would regain perfect health, but if you lost, you would die. To make an informed decision, you would want to know the chances of winning the game. The standard gamble technique is designed to estimate the risk of death that a patient would be willing to accept in a gamble for perfect health.

In this technique, subjects must choose between a health state (such as remaining in bed) and a gamble in which there is a chance of perfect health or death (see Figure 7.1). The chance of death is changed until the decision between the health state and the gamble is perceived to be about equally desirable to the subject. This process is akin to bargaining, but bargaining for perfect health. The probability decided on (p in Figure 7.1) is the utility for that health state.

For example, suppose the subject is certain that she would be willing to risk a 40 percent chance of death in exchange for the opportunity to recover from her illness but would definitely not be willing to accept a 60 percent chance of death. In other words, if the chance of death were 60 percent, she would choose the health state.

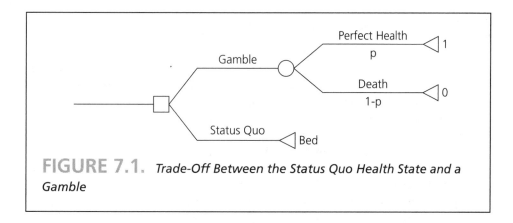

FIGURE 7.1. *Trade-Off Between the Status Quo Health State and a Gamble*

The researcher would scale the probability of death up from 40 percent until the patient is ambivalent about whether to take the gamble or remain in bed. Suppose that she finally landed on a probability of 0.55, or a 55 percent chance that she would survive. She values each year of life she lives at about 0.55 a year of perfect health.

Another technique that uses expected utility theory is called the **time trade-off** method. Here, the patient is asked how much time in poor health she would be willing to trade for perfect health. Thus, the patient has to forgo future years of life in poor health in exchange for fewer years of life in perfect health. Once the subject has decided how much time she would be willing to sacrifice for better health, the HRQL score is obtained by dividing the life expectancy in the state of illness by life expectancy in perfect health.

A final, rather primitive method involves the use of a rating scale. The subject is asked to rate the health state on a scale of 1 to 100, where 0 is the worst imaginable and 100 is the best imaginable. This is not a reference-case-compatible way of measuring HRQL but comes up a lot in cost-effectiveness cocktail parties.

Who Should Valuate HRQL?

The Panel on Cost-Effectiveness in Health and Medicine recommends that HRQL scores be determined using preference-weighted instruments that are based on a representative sample of people within society (Gold, Siegel, Russell, and Weinstein, 1996). Others believe that these scores should be obtained from people who have the disease under study. People with a disease, it is argued, know what life is like with that disease and would thus be better at valuing the corresponding quality of life than the average person would.

The problem with deriving HRQL scores from people with the disease under study is that such scores are not consistent with the societal perspective. Remember that we are interested in valuing all inputs into our cost-effectiveness analysis from the perspective of everyone in society. Deriving HRQL scores using only people with a particular disease betrays this principle. Instead, the scores should be representative of the value that the average person would assign to a particular health state (Gold, Siegel, Russell, and Weinstein, 1996).

How does a healthy person know what it is like to have a particular disease? To generate HRQL scores for health states, a sample of people go through a formal exercise in which they study different aspects of a health state. Once the person has an idea of what life might be like with the disease, the subject undergoes one of the expected utility exercises (similar to those described above) to generate an HRQL score.

When the scores are derived from a representative sample of people in a community, they are referred to as **community-derived preferences**. Again the word *preference* refers to a person's perception of what life is like in a given health state. (This perception is coaxed out with the standard gamble or time trade-off technique.)

By sampling a large group of people, we can be relatively certain to obtain the average impact of the disease, but we cannot apply these scores to individuals. Consider a study that evaluates a medication used to treat arthritis. While eccentric old writers who sit around scrawling notes in smoky cafés all day would probably prefer arthritis in their knees, runners would probably prefer to have arthritis in their hands. Moreover, both writers and runners would be affected by the arthritis in different ways. For instance, a writer earning a living from writing may see arthritis as a more severe disease than the runner would because it could lead to financial instability. Often the term *preference score* is used interchangeably with the word *utility* in cost-effectiveness analysis.

DERIVING HRQL SCORES

Much like a computer hides all of the complicated programming code behind a point-and-click interface, **preference-weighted generic instruments**—the score sheets used to generate HRQL scores—hide this methodology behind a simple survey form. One such instrument, the EuroQol, is presented in Appendix C and in Exhibit 7.1 (EuroQol Group, 1990).

These preference-weighted generic instruments may be completed using information from the medical literature. Generic HRQL instruments can also be completed by people familiar with the disease you are studying, such as patients with the disease or the doctors who are familiar with treating them (Gold, Siegel, Russell, and Weinstein, 1996). Such a range of people can fill them out and get comparable scores because the categories are quite broad. Most people would agree that someone with a cold has some discomfort but not severe discomfort. For this reason too, it's not necessary to obtain a large sample of people to fill these out. Three doctors or three patients ought to do if the condition you are evaluating is relatively straightforward.

Once the instrument is completed, the researcher inputs the responses into a simple formula that produces an HRQL score suitable for use in a reference case cost-effectiveness analysis. This is discussed in the next section.

In the following sections, we examine how to obtain scores using preference-weighted generic instruments, how to use scores derived from published lists, and how to use HRQL scores in nonreference case measures, such as the disability-adjusted life year (DALY).

EXHIBIT 7.1. EuroQol 5D Health Domains

Mobility
I have no problems in walking about ☐
I have some problems in walking about ☐
I am confined to bed ☐

Self-Care
I have no problems with self-care ☐
I have some problems washing or dressing myself ☐
I am unable to wash or dress myself ☐

Usual Activities (*e.g., work, study, housework, family, or leisure activities*)
I have no problems with performing my usual activities ☐
I have some problems with performing my usual activities ☐
I am unable to perform my usual activities ☐

Pain/Discomfort
I have no pain or discomfort ☐
I have moderate pain or discomfort ☐
I have extreme pain or discomfort ☐

Anxiety/Depression
I am not anxious or depressed ☐
I am moderately anxious or depressed ☐
I am extremely anxious or depressed ☐

Very large research efforts sometimes also generate scores by taking a sample of subjects through a series of exercises based on expected utility theory (for example, the standard gamble or time trade-off) so that they can generate HRQL scores from scratch.

Using Preference-Weighted Generic Instruments

Preference-weighted generic instruments are often used in cost-effectiveness analysis because the process of determining community-derived HRQL scores is costly and time-consuming (Gold, Siegel, Russell, and Weinstein, 1996). Each preference-weighted generic instrument has its strengths and weaknesses. Examples are the Quality of Well-Being (QWB) scale, the Health Utility Index, and the EuroQol.

Recall that these instruments may be used to convert responses from physicians or patients who have experience with the disease under study into HRQL scores that estimate preferences derived from a representative community sample. Alternatively, researchers can sometimes obtain information about the disease from the medical literature and then use this information to fill in the blanks of a preference-weighted generic instrument. In other words, preference-weighted generic instruments are essentially tools that translate survey responses into HRQL scores derived from a large, representative community sample of people who have gone through exercises grounded in expected utility theory.

Again, to reiterate, each of these scores derived from the community sample is associated with a particular aspect of a given health state (as in Exhibit 7.1). Each of these responses is referred to as a **dimension** (also known as an **attribute** or **domain**). One example of a dimension is "depressed versus happy." Another is whether someone can get around. The dimensions are broken into levels (for example, "no problem," "some problem," or "severe problems). Preference-weighted generic instruments are therefore more generally called **multiattribute health status classification systems**, because they combine different levels of many different attributes of a given disease into a single HRQL score (Drummond, O'Brien, Stoddart, and Torrance, 2005).

So what's the difference between these and a health state? *Health state* is a more general term. For instance, being able to walk is a health state, but so is just being alive. We wouldn't typically speak of being alive as a health dimension.

The dimensions captured by an instrument can represent aspects of a disease beyond the biological symptoms the disease causes. For instance, diabetes can cause blindness or the inability to walk. These conditions may in turn affect the person's ability to function in society and may place strains on his or her relationships with others. Blindness, the inability to walk, a person's ability to function in society, a person's ability to relate to others, and a person's ability to work are all examples of health dimensions.

Let's see how this might play out in one example. Consider the man with moderately severe diabetes. He has numbness in the feet and some problems walking but can still take care of himself. He has intermittent pain and moderate discomfort from intestinal manifestations of the disease. Because he is not dependent on others, the disease has not greatly affected his autonomy, and he does not feel anxious or depressed as a result. Knowing this, filling out the instrument (Exhibit 7.1) becomes merely a matter of checking off the boxes.

TIPS AND TRICKS

Culture influences the way that we think about health states and therefore affects the results of exercises such as the time trade-off or standard gamble. For this reason, the preference scores used in preference-weighted generic instruments vary from country to country. The EuroQol contains preference weights from a number of countries, so translating scores requires little more than applying a different scoring formula.

In this instance, the man has some trouble walking about, so we might check the second box in Exhibit 7.1 under Mobility. He does not have any problems with self-care, so we might check the first box there. We weren't given any information about his ability to perform his usual activities. If his usual activities involve sitting in front of the television set, then we might check the first box. But most people would be hampered by the foot numbness and intermittent pain to limit usual activities, so we might check the second box. On the Pain/Discomfort scale, you would probably give him a moderate rating. The rating for Anxiety/Depression is tricky. Some folks become depressed by the onset of chronic disease, while others shrug it off. Most adapt fairly well over time, though, so we might want to check the "I am not anxious or depressed" box.

Probably most students provided with this information would check off a similar pattern of boxes, even though the information about usual activities was incomplete. Again, this is the beauty of these instruments; they allow enough leeway that there is a low likelihood that two people would generate radically different scores when given a particular scenario.

Let's now score that man's HRQL using U.S. weights (see Appendix C for the weights). To obtain the HRQL score for him using the EuroQol, we subtract the weights for each score from 1.0. Recall that the scores are as follows: Mobility = 2, Self Care = 1, Usual Activities = 2, Pain/Discomfort = 2, Anxiety/Depression = 1. Checking these against the U.S. weights in Appendix C, we see that the respective weights are Mobility = 0.146, Self Care = 0, Usual Activities = 0.14, Pain/Discomfort = 0.173, and Anxiety/Depression = 0. The sum of all of these weights is 0.459. To obtain the EuroQol score, we subtract this number from 1.0 to obtain an HRQL score of 0.541.

What if you don't have a tidy case scenario like this one? In most cases, we will have a decision analysis model that looks something like the one in Figure 7.2. Suppose that we wish to model the effects of a diabetes treatment on modulating the severity of the disease. In this model, subjects with diabetes are classified into three states: mild, moderate, and severe. At the end of the year, subjects in the Mild branch are returned

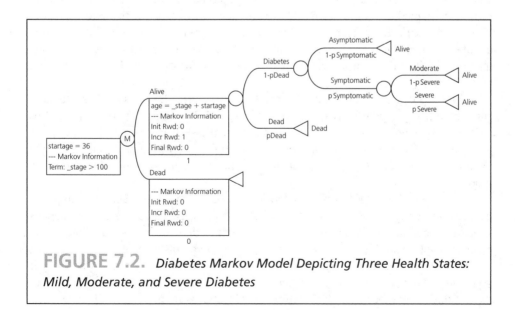

FIGURE 7.2. *Diabetes Markov Model Depicting Three Health States: Mild, Moderate, and Severe Diabetes*

to the Alive branch, where they are exposed to a risk of death, remaining in the Mild category, or progressing to the Moderate or Severe category.

Were we to assign HRQL scores to this model, we would need three scores: (1) asymptomatic, (2) moderate diabetes, and (3) severe diabetes. We have to decide what asymptomatic/mild, moderate, and severe diabetes look like. To estimate the HRQL of each severity level of diabetes using the EuroQol, we could turn to an endocrinologist who sees the disease all the time. Most endocrinologists would check the top box for each dimension of mild diabetes because it does not produce any symptoms. There might be some disagreement as to what moderate or severe diabetes looks like, but if we asked five to six endocrinologists, we would probably get a good idea of what the HRQL score for these health states looks like as well.

TIPS AND TRICKS

By now you should have a rough idea of how many professionals you might need to consult to obtain your HRQL score. If the disease is straightforward, a few will do. If it is not, you'll need a few more. If three professionals come up with the same score, you are probably good to go. But if the scores differ, you'll probably need a larger sample. This isn't a problem if the researcher is able to obtain information on health states from the medical literature.

You probably sense that using the EuroQol to score this disease will provide a rough or shotgun approach to deriving a score. Since diabetes mostly affects self-care, mobility, and ability to perform usual activities while potentially causing anxiety and depression, this is probably a good instrument for scoring this disease. However, if we wanted to derive the HRQL of someone with kleptomania, we probably wouldn't get very far with the EuroQol; we would have only a gauge of how much anxiety the condition was causing the average kleptomaniac. For this reason, it is a good idea to think about the dimensions of one's HRQL that are affected by the disease under study and try to match it to the instruments available as best as one can (Gold, Siegel, Russell, and Weinstein, 1996).

Let us consider another example. The Quality of Well-Being (QWB) scale measures mobility, physical activity, social activity, and the effect of various symptoms such as fatigue on HRQL (Kaplan and Anderson, 1988). If we were to use the QWB to obtain an HRQL score for diabetes, we would capture the impact diabetes might have on the subject's social life, but the instrument would still miss his depressed mood.

Fortunately, both the EuroQol and QWB are based on a representative sample of people's preferences for disease states. Because preferences reflect many people's subjective perception of what life would be like with a disease, it is not absolutely necessary to capture all dimensions of a disease in any given instrument.

Why? Consider the example of the runner and the writer with arthritis. Even if you didn't have a questionnaire that included mobility limitations, the plight of each of these folks would be partially captured in (1) ability to perform daily activities, (2) anxiety and depression, and (3) pain and discomfort. Obviously you will be able to get a better-specified score with mobility in the instrument, but you'll still get some idea of the person's HRQL score with these other three dimensions.

Generating HRQL for Acute Conditions

In the previous example, we saw how we might score diabetes using a case scenario or the input of an endocrinologist. In that example, we saw that a subject's HRQL was determined by the severity of disease from one year to the next. Now let's look at how the EuroQol might be used to generate an HRQL score for influenza (a condition that lasts for only five days) using data from the medical literature.

This example uses rounded data from Keech, Scott, and Ryan (1998), who estimate that subjects with the flu are confined to bed for two days, require one day of caregiver support, and miss 3 days of work on average. Now let us assume that on days 1, 4, and 5, most patients with influenza-like illness are able to get around but they are confined to bed on days 2 through 3. Let us assume that people generally have some self-care difficulties on day 3 and miss work on days 2 through 4. We'll pretend that this is an English patient and apply U.K. weights.

To obtain an HRQL score for any given day, subtract the preference weight values in Table 7.1 from 1.0. For instance, we see that on day 2, the person's mobility severity rating is 3 (confined to bed), which is associated with a score of 0.314.

TABLE 7.1. **Example of How an HRQL Score for Influenza Illness May Be Derived Using the EuroQol**

	Day 1 (No Symptoms)	Day 2 (Symptoms Begin)	Day 3 (Most Severe)	Day 4 (Improving)	Day 5 (Feels Better)
Mobility	1 (0.000)	3 (0.314)	3 (0.314)	1 (0.000)	1 (0.000)
Self-care	1 (0.000)	1 (0.000)	2 (0.104)	1 (0.000)	1 (0.000)
Usual activity	1 (0.000)	3 (0.094)	3 (0.094)	3 (0.094)	1 (0.000)
Pain	1 (0.000)	1 (0.000)	1 (0.000)	1 (0.000)	1 (0.000)
Anxiety/depression	1 (0.000)	1 (0.000)	1 (0.000)	1 (0.000)	1 (0.000)
Score for day	1	0.511	0.407	0.825	1

Note: The severity rating for each day and each dimension in the EuroQol is presented alongside weights for each state. For instance, on day 2, influenza is given a mobility rating of 3, and the weight for this mobility rating is 0.314.

Looking at Table 7.1, we see that in addition to a mobility rating of 3, the person has a usual activity rating of 3 on day 2, which is associated with a weight of 0.094. In this example, we are applying U.K. weights. Whenever the severity rating (or level) is more than 1, we also have to subtract 0.081 from the score in the U.K. Thus, the person's total score for the day using U.K. weights and the U.K. formula is $1.0 - 0.314 - 0.094 - 0.081 = 0.511$.

TIPS AND TRICKS

The only trick to calculating the HRQL score using this particular instrument in the United Kingdom is that a constant value (0.081) is used to adjust the overall score. This must be applied whenever the person is in less than perfect health. (The technical reason is that the value is obtained using linear regression and therefore has an intercept, or constant value.) In the United States, no constant value is used (Shaw, Johnson, and Coons, 2005), so we simply subtract the weights from 1.0. For country-specific weights, see Appendix C. Values for other countries must be looked up in the medical literature.

The mean HRQL over the 5 days spent with the flu is calculated by averaging across all days (adding up all of the values and dividing by 5), yielding a score of 0.75. If we were to apply the same values to the QWB scale, we would obtain an HRQL score of 0.61. The scores differ between these instruments for a number of reasons. First, the weights are based on a different community sample of people. Second, each instrument captures different dimensions of the disease. The QWB scale allows us to capture specific symptoms of influenza, such as coughing and wheezing, so it may afford more specificity. Finally, each is based on a different method for estimating HRQL (Gold and Muennig, 2002).

TIPS AND TRICKS

Here we applied HRQL scores to an acute illness: influenza virus infection. We got creative by averaging the scores across various days of illness. This serves to illustrate how HRQL can change throughout the course of illness. However, in reality, HRQL scores are not designed to be applied to acute infectious diseases. Unfortunately, there is no alternative system for acute illness, so we have to make do with these scores.

HRQL Scores Generated from Large Health Surveys

It is also possible to use large national health surveys that contain questions similar to those in preference-weighted generic instruments to generate complete lists of HRQL scores for different diseases. This is especially useful for estimating the average HRQL for people with and without a disease because it provides a national average. It also comes in handy when estimating the overall HRQL associated with a risk factor for multiple diseases. For instance, the MEPS has been used to estimate the HRQL of people with and without health insurance and the HRQL of people with varying levels of income (Muennig, Franks, and Gold, 2005; Muennig and others, 2005).

How does this work? The mean responses from the national survey in question are essentially matched to responses on the generic instrument. The MEPS even contains a variable with each subject's HRQL score, so there is no need to do all of the matching yourself. Of course, using a national dataset to calculate an HRQL score requires familiarity with the use of datasets and a statistical software package.

OTHER CONSIDERATIONS AND REMINDERS

When beginning cost-effectiveness researchers first roll up their sleeves and get to work on a cost-effectiveness analysis, they often derive their HRQL score without really considering what it means. In this section, I briefly review a few of the most commonly overlooked contributors to HRQL.

Effect of Age on HRQL

In general, younger people tend to think about health very differently from older people. An elderly person may not place a high value on sexual function, for example, but a younger person almost certainly will. Moreover, because younger people are on average in better health than older people, they tend to have higher average HRQL scores and tend to place very different values on different health states.

Effect of Disease Stage on HRQL

It is important to obtain HRQL scores specific to different stages of a disease (Figure 7.1). For instance, adult-onset diabetes is usually asymptomatic in its early stages; however, various aspects of a diabetic's health tend to deteriorate over time. These changes include the loss of sensation in limbs, loss of vision, repeated hospitalizations, and a number of other problems. These conditions also tend to develop concurrent with one another, complicating the person's overall health status.

Effect of an Intervention on HRQL

If diabetes is appropriately managed, the likelihood of developing future complications is reduced, and thus the general health status of treated persons will be improved relative to those who are untreated. However, the treatment itself can be associated with side effects that can have an impact on a person's health.

Because a cost-effectiveness analysis must evaluate the differences between people who have and have not received a particular intervention, such as medications used to treat diabetes mellitus, scores must be estimated for subjects in the intervention and nonintervention groups. The trick thus becomes deciding how to measure how much the treatment slows the progression of the disease relative to no treatment and how much harm the treatment is itself causing. Clearly this kind of nuanced analysis must be conducted with the input of endocrinologists and guided by the medical literature.

Use of HRQL Scores in Diverse Populations

Health-related quality-of-life scores for a disease may be different for men and women, persons of different social classes, and other groups. Some care should be taken when applying HRQL scores to a group that differs demographically from the general population (Lubetkin, Jia, Franks, and Gold, 2005).

USING DISABILITY-ADJUSTED LIFE YEARS

One last method that should be mentioned, but is not accepted by many health economists, is the practice of deriving preference scores from experts rather than a representative community sample. The scores associated with the DALY were derived using experts in part because it was necessary to generate scores for many conditions, and in part because the scores were to be applied to people in distinct geographical regions of the world (Murray and Lopez, 1996).

The disability-adjusted life year is a QALY in reverse: it measures the years of healthy life lost to disease rather than the years of healthy life gained by an intervention. Because of this, the HRQL scores associated with the DALY vary on a scale where 0 is equal to perfect health and 1 is equal to death (the opposite of HRQL scores associated with QALYs). To convert a DALY score into a standard HRQL score, the score must be subtracted from 1.0.

Recall that generic preference-weighted instruments are based on community-generated preference weights. If a physician fills out the instrument, therefore, the physician's responses are translated into community weights. In the DALY, health professionals generate the weights themselves. This presents a number of problems (Gold, Siegel, Russell, and Weinstein, 1996). For example, physicians may be likely to overrate the physical aspects of an illness but underrate the psychological aspects. These scores are therefore not technically QALY compatible—and for good reason: the DALY can actually change the ranking of some diseases in a league table relative to QALY-compatible measures (Gold and Muennig, 2002). As we will see in the next chapter, cost-effectiveness analyses that do use the DALY must modify the methods used slightly because this measure was designed for burden-of-disease analysis rather than cost-effectiveness analysis.

CHAPTER

8

CALCULATING QALYs

OVERVIEW

THIS CHAPTER demonstrates various approaches to calculating QALYs. Each approach provides a unique perspective on what QALYs are, how they are used, and how they are calculated. We call these methods (1) the life table method, (2) the Markov method, and (3) the summation method.

In the life table method, a spreadsheet is used to calculate the number of deaths and person-years remaining in a hypothetical cohort, as we did in Chapter Six. These person-years are then adjusted for HRQL to obtain the total QALYs lived (Erickson, Wilson, and Shannon, 1995; Muennig and Gold, 2002). In the Markov method, subjects in a hypothetical cohort gain 1 QALY for each year they remain alive. We also saw how this worked in Chapter Six but used life years rather than QALYs. The summation method is used when we have concrete information on the changes in life years and HRQL associated with an intervention already on hand (Drummond, O'Brien, Stoddart, and Torrance, 2005).

We also discuss the disability-adjusted life year (DALY), which is often used in studies within developing countries or studies comparing the burden of disease among nations. While a QALY is a year of perfect health gained, a DALY is a year of perfect health lost to disease (Murray and Lopez, 1996). Those who use DALYs are not simply a bunch of pessimistic health economists. Rather, this inverted definition arises from how DALYs are used (typically to capture the burden of disease) and how they are calculated.

117

We begin by exploring how to calculate the incremental number of QALYs gained by summation. We demonstrate how to calculate QALYs using the life table method and then move on to a worked example using Markov models. The last bit will be dedicated to the DALY.

■ ■ ■

USING THE SUMMATION METHOD

Let's go a few months into the future. You have finished reading this book, and a researcher wants to hire you to help her team perform a cost-effectiveness analysis of a new treatment for a tropical disease, leishmaniasis, in sub-Saharan Africa.

They've provided you with five years of follow-up data from a randomized controlled trial. You've calculated the change in costs, but you need to figure out how this treatment has changed the quality and quantity of life for these subjects over this five-year period.

The summation method is most often used when gains in life expectancy and HRQL are more or less identifiable. This situation is sometimes encountered in economic evaluations conducted in developing countries. It's also quite useful for illustrating the basic concepts behind QALYs (Drummond, O'Brien, Stoddart, and Torrance, 2005).

Suppose that the new treatment for leishmaniasis has an unknown impact on the overall quality of life but improves life expectancy by one year over the five-year span of the study and that the average person with the disease has a three-year life expectancy. We consult the literature and find that the average HRQL of people with leishmaniasis is 0.5 and the average untreated life expectancy is three years. Thus, each year that the subjects are alive, they gain 0.5 QALYs. Assuming that the treatment prolongs life but produces no improvement in HRQL, the two interventions (treatment versus no treatment) would accrue the following QALYs:

$$\begin{aligned} \text{Treatment:} \quad & 0.5 + 0.5 + 0.5 + 0.5 = 2 \text{ QALYs} \\ \text{No treatment:} \quad & 0.5 + 0.5 + 0.5 + 0 \;\; = 1.5 \text{ QALYs} \end{aligned} \qquad (8.1)$$

The total number of QALYs gained by treatment is 2 QALYs − 1.5 QALYs = 0.5 QALYs. Had we not adjusted for HRQL, the gain would have been 4 years − 3 years = 1 year.

Now suppose that we estimate the impact of the treatment on various health states and calculate changes in HRQL using a preference-weighted instrument. If we know that the mean HRQL of treated people is 0.6 and the mean HRQL of untreated people is 0.5, then we can also account for the ability of the drug to improve one's quality of life:

$$\begin{aligned} \text{Treatment:} \quad & 0.6 + 0.6 + 0.6 + 0.6 = 2.4 \text{ QALYs} \\ \text{No treatment:} \quad & 0.5 + 0.5 + 0.5 + 0 \;\; = 1.5 \text{ QALYs} \end{aligned} \qquad (8.2)$$

The total number of QALYs gained by treatment is 2.4 − 1.5 = 0.9.

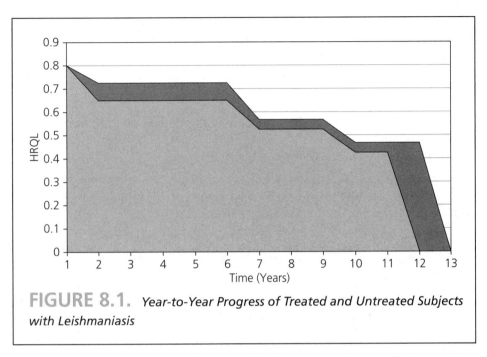

FIGURE 8.1. *Year-to-Year Progress of Treated and Untreated Subjects with Leishmaniasis*

Note: The light area represents untreated patients and the dark area treated patients. The incremental gain in QALYs is the difference between the dark area and light area.

Now let us go one step further still and consider the lifetime health pathway for people with this disease. Suppose that a different group of researchers managed to obtain year-to-year data on the subjects' specific HRQL with this disease. They also intervened at an earlier stage of disease, so the cohort lived longer, and followed them over many years. The researchers manage to plot the health status in the number of deaths over time of subjects in their cohort (Figure 8.1). The light-shaded curve in the figure represents their quality-adjusted life expectancy (QALE) if untreated, and the dark-shaded curve represents their average QALE if treated. In this case, the incremental gain in QALYs is equal to the area under the dark shaded curve minus the area under the light shaded curve. Said another way, it is equal to $QALE_{Treated} - QALE_{Untreated}$.

We see too that the average treated person in this graph lived twelve years and the average untreated person thirteen years. However, the total QALYs gained differ substantially because the treated group has a higher HRQL. Keep this image in your head; it will come in handy to understand how more complex methods work.

USING THE LIFE TABLE METHOD

Life expectancy may be calculated using a **standard life table** or an **abridged life table** (Anderson, 1999). A standard life table calculates life expectancy for a group of people based on the mortality rate over one-year age intervals, and an abridged life table uses five-year (or longer) age intervals. Thus, although an abridged life table is easier to construct, a standard life table is slightly more accurate. Appendix B contains abridged life tables and quality-adjusted life tables for the U.S. population for 2003.

Pull up the spreadsheet we used in Chapter Six containing person-years. (If you are following along without the spreadsheet, Table 6.5 is renamed Table 8.1 and presented below.)

TABLE 8.1.   **Total Person-Years Lived by the Cohort of 1 Million 15 Year Olds**

Age	Alive (1)	All Deaths (2)	Person-Years (Col. 1 − Col. 2 × 0.5) (3)
15	1,000,000	407	999,797
16	999,593	575	999,306
17	999,018	683	998,677
18	998,335	728	997,971
19	997,607	734	997,240
20	996,873	898	996,424
. . .	. . .	. . .	. . .
95	29,011	11,589	23,217
96	17,422	8,754	13,045
97	8,668	3,989	6,674
98	4,679	1,234	4,062
99	3,445	2,038	2,426
100	1,407	664	1,075
Total	64,169,845		63,670,217

TIPS AND TRICKS

For the completed exercise, see Table 8.1 at http://www.pceo.org/learn.html.

Let's begin by calculating life expectancy at each age in Table 8.1. To do this, first sum up the total person-years lived in the cohort starting with the first cell at the bottom of column 3. Thus, we add the number of person-years lived by 100 year olds (1,075) to the number lived by 99 year olds (2,426) in the age 99 cell of column 3 to obtain the cumulative total person-years by age 99 (1,075 + 2,426 = 3,502). We then repeat this process across all ages as in column 4 of Table 8.2.

Finally, to calculate life expectancy at each age, we divide the number of subjects alive at the start of any given age (column 1) interval by the cumulative total person-years (column 4) up to that age (see Table 8.3). Recall that by dividing the total number of years lived by the total number of people that lived them yields the mean number of years lived per person.

You just learned how to build a life table. In the first part of Chapter Six, you learned how to work with abridged data. In the second part, you learned how to calculate the total person-years and the life expectancy using year-to-year data. Here, we combine these two concepts. Table 8.4 is an abridged life table for 2003.

In this table, we begin with the probability of dying within any age group, which is essentially the mortality rate for that age group (column 1). This rate is obtained using national mortality data (Hoyert, Kung, and Smith, 2005). We then apply this mortality rate to a hypothetical cohort of 100,000 newborn babies (column 2) to obtain the total number of deaths in each age interval (column 3). (In other words, column 3 is column 1 times column 2.) Using these data, we estimate the total person-years in the interval, which you are now familiar with (column 4). Summing column 4 data by age interval, we obtain the total person-years lived by the cohort up to that age. And finally, the total person-years in the cohort divided by the number of subjects at the start (in this case 100,000 persons) is equal to the life expectancy of the cohort (column 5).

TIPS AND TRICKS

Recall from Chapter Six that the number of person-years is equal to the number alive at the beginning of the age interval plus one-half of the deaths in that interval.

Quality-Adjusted Life Expectancy

Quality-adjusted life expectancy (QALE) is the number of years of perfect health one can expect to live at birth. You get this number by multiplying the total person-years within an age interval by the age-specific HRQL score for that age interval (see Table 8.5).

In Table 8.5, we see that the people in the first year had an HRQL of 0.95. The product of the HRQL score and the person-years in the age interval yields the total QALYs lived by the cohort in that age interval. If we sum the total QALYs lived in each age interval across all intervals, we get the total QALYs lived by the cohort. Once again, we divide by the 100,000 people at the start of the cohort to get QALE.

TABLE 8.2. **Sum of Person-Years Across Age Groups for the Cohort of 1 Million 15 Year Olds**

Column	1	2	3	4
				Cumulative Person-Years Sum of Col. 3 values from
Age	Alive	All Deaths	Person-Years Col. 1 − Col. 2 × 0.5	bottom
15	1,000,000	407	999,797	63,670,217
16	999,593	575	999,306	62,670,421
17	999,018	683	998,677	61,671,115
18	998,335	728	997,971	60,672,439
19	997,607	734	997,240	59,674,468
20	996,873	898	996,424	58,677,228
. . .	. . .	. . .	. . .	. . .
95	29,011	11,589	23,217	50,500
96	17,422	8,754	13,045	27,283
97	8,668	3,989	6,674	14,238
98	4,679	1,234	4,062	7,564
99	3,445	2,038	2,426	3,501	⟵ 1,075 + 2,426
100	1,407	664	1,075	1,075

TABLE 8.3. **Calculating Life Expectancy at a Given Age**

Age	Alive (1)	All Deaths (2)	Person-Years (Col. 1 − Col. 2 × 0.5) (3)	Cumulative Person-Years (Sum of Col. 3 Values from Bottom) (4)	Life Expectancy (Col. 4/Col. 1) (5)
15	1,000,000	407	999,797	63,670,217	63.67
16	999,593	575	999,306	62,670,421	62.70
17	999,018	683	998,677	61,671,115	61.73
18	998,335	728	997,971	60,672,439	60.77
19	997,607	734	997,240	59,674,468	59.82
20	996,873	898	996,424	58,677,228	58.86
...	...	...	...	...	...
95	29,011	11,589	23,217	50,500	1.74
96	17,422	8,754	13,045	27,283	1.57
97	8,668	3,989	6,674	14,238	1.64
98	4,679	1,234	4,062	7,564	1.62
99	3,445	2,038	2,426	3,501	1.02
100	1,407	664	1,075	1,075	0.76

Note: Life expectancy at any age is calculated by the total alive at that age by the cumulative person-years lived at that age.

TABLE 8.4. Abridged Life Table for 2003

Age	Probability of Dying Between Ages X and $X + N$ (1)	Number Surviving to Age X (2)	Number Dying Between Ages X and $X + N$ (Col. 1 × Col. 2) (3)	Person-Years Lived Between Ages X and $X + N$ (Col. 2 − Col. 3 × 0.5) (4)	Total Number of Person-Years Lived Above Age X (Sum of Col. 4 Values) (5)	Expectancy of Life at Age X (Col. 5 / Col. 2) (6)
0–1	0.006865	100,000	687	99,394	7,748,865	77.5
1–5	0.001252	99,313	124	396,962	7,649,471	77.0
5–10	0.000734	99,189	73	495,756	7,252,510	73.1
10–15	0.000956	99,116	95	495,369	6,756,754	68.2
15–20	0.003317	99,022	328	494,435	6,261,385	63.2
20–25	0.004806	98,693	474	492,277	5,766,950	58.4
25–30	0.004751	98,219	467	489,938	5,274,672	53.7
30–35	0.005541	97,752	542	487,457	4,784,734	48.9
35–40	0.007886	97,210	767	484,249	4,297,277	44.2

Age					
40–45	0.011992	96,444	1,157	479,513	3,813,027	39.5
45–50	0.017862	95,287	1,702	472,435	3,333,515	35.0
50–55	0.025653	93,585	2,401	462,242	2,861,080	30.6
55–60	0.037558	91,185	3,425	447,912	2,398,838	26.3
60–65	0.058021	87,760	5,092	426,797	1,950,925	22.2
65–70	0.086287	82,668	7,133	396,471	1,524,128	18.4
70–75	0.130072	75,535	9,825	354,252	1,127,657	14.9
75–80	0.197364	65,710	12,969	297,321	773,405	11.8
80–85	0.298685	52,741	15,753	224,973	476,084	9.0
85–90	0.423047	36,988	15,648	145,292	251,112	6.8
90–95	0.579341	21,340	12,363	73,760	105,820	5.0
95–100	0.736793	8,977	6,614	26,017	32,060	3.6
100 and over	1.000000	2,363	2,363	6,044	6,044	2.6

TABLE 8.5. A Quality-Adjusted Life Table

Age	Probability of Dying Between Ages X and X + N (1)	Number Surviving to Age X (2)	Number Dying Between Ages X and X + N (Col. 1 × Col. 2) (3)	Person-Years Lived Between Ages X and X + N (Col. 2 − Col. 3 × 0.5) (4)	HRQL Score (Obtained from MEPS) (5)[a]	Quality-Adjusted Person-Years Lived Between X and X + N (Col. 4 × Col. 5) (6)	Total Quality-Adjusted Number of Person-Years Lived Above Age X (Sum of Col. 6 Values) (7)	Quality-Adjusted Expectancy of Life at Age X (Col. 7/ Col. 2) (8)
0–1	0.006865	100,000	687	99,394	0.95	94,402	6,522,725	65.2
1–5	0.001252	99,313	124	396,962	0.94	374,988	6,428,323	64.7
5–10	0.000734	99,189	73	495,756	0.93	458,985	6,053,335	61.0
10–15	0.000956	99,116	95	495,369	0.92	458,118	5,594,350	56.4
15–20	0.003317	99,022	328	494,435	0.90	443,385	5,136,233	51.9
20–25	0.004806	98,693	474	492,277	0.89	438,151	4,692,847	47.5
25–30	0.004751	98,219	467	489,938	0.89	436,069	4,254,696	43.3

30–35	0.005541	97,752	542	487,457	0.84	407,067	3,818,627	39.1
35–40	0.007886	97,210	767	484,249	0.84	404,388	3,411,560	35.1
40–45	0.011992	96,444	1,157	479,513	0.84	400,432	3,007,172	31.2
45–50	0.017862	95,287	1,702	472,435	0.84	394,522	2,606,740	27.4
50–55	0.025653	93,585	2,401	462,242	0.79	365,318	2,212,218	23.6
55–60	0.037558	91,185	3,425	447,912	0.79	353,992	1,846,900	20.3
60–65	0.058021	87,760	5,092	426,797	0.79	337,305	1,492,908	17.0
65–70	0.086287	82,668	7,133	396,471	0.79	313,338	1,155,602	14.0
70–75	0.130072	75,535	9,825	354,252	0.76	267,999	842,265	11.2

[a]Values for those under 18 were not available in the MEPS, and were obtained using predictive linear regression.

TIPS AND TRICKS

To follow along, download example 8.2 from http://www.pceo.org/learn.html.

Of course, a person's QALE changes when disease is present; disease can affect health (and thus HRQL) or life expectancy, or both. It also changes when different medical interventions are administered. Like disease, health interventions have an effect on the quality and quantity of life. The number of QALYs gained when a health intervention is implemented is calculated using the equation

$$\text{QALE}_{\text{intervention 1}} - \text{QALE}_{\text{intervention 2}} \qquad (8.3)$$

where intervention 1 is the more effective intervention.

How do we go about this? Simple. We just estimate the change in life expectancy and the change in HRQL associated with an intervention, calculate QALE with and without the intervention, and voilá!

Now think back to Figure 8.1. This figure showed that the health pathways between people given an intervention and people not given an intervention differ from year-to-year. Here, we see that a quality-adjusted life table does precisely that.

EXERCISES 1 TO 4

To complete these exercises, you'll need to download the 2003 QALE calculator from http://www.pceo.org/learn.html.

1. Desperate for a job out of public health school, you have taken a job with a health foods company. It has produced a new product called Super Holistic Chakra Enhancer, which it claims reduces mortality by 50 percent. It has asked you to translate this miraculous effect into life years gained. You shrug your shoulders and set to the calculations. What number do you give for the total years gained by an infant given this formula for the rest of his or her life? Tip: Enter the risk ratio into the column labeled "crude risk ratio," and see how the overall life expectancy changes.

2. You quit your job working on Super Holistic Chakra Enhancer and decide to join a group working on the cost-effectiveness of a new drug to lower blood sugar in diabetics. The target audience has a mean age of disease onset of 60 years. You wish to know how the drug compares to the current practice. You find that the average diabetic over age 60 is at 10 percent greater annual risk of mortality than the average person in the United States. The new drug has been shown to have a risk ratio of 0.95 compared to current practice among diabetics. How many years of life will be gained on average? Hint: Be sure to enter risk ratios starting at age 60 in the table.

3. Your next step is to calculate the gain in QALE. You go to the Medical Expenditure Panel survey linked to mortality data and find that the mean HRQL for people over age 60 is 0.7. Your team finds that there is a 10 percent improvement in HRQL. How many QALYs are gained when this new treatment is consistently given to diabetics?

4. Just for fun, let's see what your life expectancy is relative to the average person in your country. If you are from the United States, use the life table provided. Otherwise you can build your own life table by copying age-specific mortality probabilities from a life table from your ministry of health (any search engine should get you there). Assuming you are on your way to some graduate degree, here is a rough indicator of your risk of death at any given age: (1) If you are from a country with very few college-educated people, give yourself a risk ratio of about 0.5 beginning at your current age. (2) If you are from a country with a high number of college-educated people (for example, the United States, Japan, countries in Europe, Cuba), give yourself a risk ratio of about 0.65. (This is lower because the average person is somewhat more likely to have a college or graduate degree, putting him or her closer to you.) Note that the answer to this exercise is age and country dependent, so there is no answer provided in the key.

Using Markov Models to Calculate QALE

In Chapter Six, you saw that life expectancy is calculated in a Markov model by granting survivors one year of life. To calculate QALE, we simply substitute the one-year gain every year with the age-specific HRQL score.

TIPS AND TRICKS

If you have not yet worked through the examples in the laboratory workbook, do so now. It will help you better understand the concepts presented here.

Recall that every time the tree cycles, we gain one year of life expectancy (Incr Rwd = 1) and that the annual risk of death is obtained from a life table. In Figure 8.2, this is represented as tDead[_stage]. In this diagram, [_stage] indicates how many cycles have been completed. So when the subject is 10 years of age, _stage = 10. A

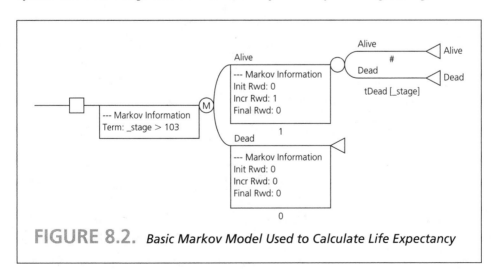

FIGURE 8.2. *Basic Markov Model Used to Calculate Life Expectancy*

subject who has an HRQL of 0.9 rather than 1.0 would have lived 9 QALYs over these 10 cycles.

Let's take this to the next level to see how we might calculate the QALYs gained by a particular intervention using Markov models. Suppose that you are comparing two surgical treatments for a congenital heart valve defect. This defect affects new-borns but can be corrected using one of these two procedures at birth.

The first procedure is called the Filmore procedure (after Ignacious Danenhousen Filmore) and does a pretty good job of fixing the problem at no initial risk to the infant to speak of. However, each year, the person will be at a 25 percent increased risk of mortality due to the incomplete nature of this surgical technique.

Recently Ludviga Elmore Reinkenshein modified the Filmore procedure so that it completely fixes the heart defect. However, she patented her surgical technique, so it's expensive, requiring the hospital to pay $10,000 to her every time it's used. Let's first look at these two procedures in terms of effectiveness alone.

We know that babies who receive the Reinkenshein procedure have an approximately normal life expectancy. Those who receive the Filmore procedure will be at

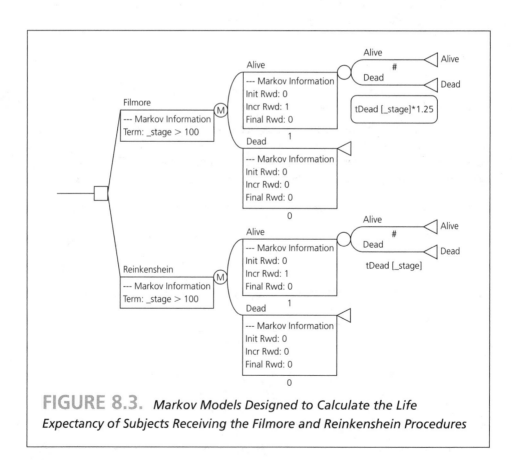

FIGURE 8.3. *Markov Models Designed to Calculate the Life Expectancy of Subjects Receiving the Filmore and Reinkenshein Procedures*

25 percent increased risk of death. Therefore, if tDead[_stage] in Figure 8.2 reflects the mean life expectancy in the United States, the risk of death among those receiving the Filmore procedure is simply 1.25 × the age-specific mortality rate. (In other words, the age-specific mortality rate increased by 25 percent.) This change can be seen in the top portion of Figure 8.3. Notice that tDead[_stage] is multiplied by 1.25 to reflect the higher mortality in this group.

Now let's add a measure of HRQL to each arm. Suppose that we take a group of patients living with the Filmore procedure and a group living with the Reinkenshein procedure and have them fill out the EuroQol. We find that those with the Filmore procedure have an average HRQL of 0.8, and those who have the Reinkenshein procedure have an average HRQL of 0.85. To calculate the difference in QALE, we give subjects with the Filmore procedure a gain of 0.8 for every year that they lived and those who had the Reinkenshein procedure a gain of 0.85 (Figure 8.4).

Now, let's see what happens when we calculate the QALE of each competing alternative (Figure 8.5). Here we see that greedy Ludviga's procedure does result in a significantly longer QALE—about seven years of additional life lived in perfect health. The next logical question is: Is this worth the extra cost?

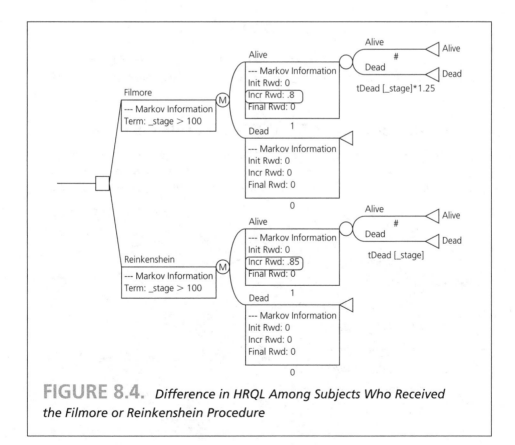

FIGURE 8.4. *Difference in HRQL Among Subjects Who Received the Filmore or Reinkenshein Procedure*

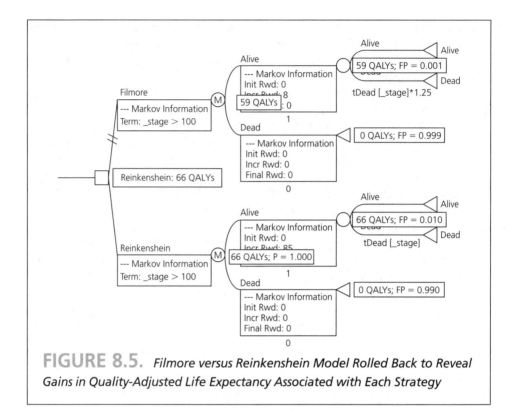

FIGURE 8.5. *Filmore versus Reinkenshein Model Rolled Back to Reveal Gains in Quality-Adjusted Life Expectancy Associated with Each Strategy*

CALCULATING INCREMENTAL COST-EFFECTIVENESS

Now we add cost differences to the model and show how a Markov model calculates incremental cost-effectiveness ratios. Let's say that we know that each procedure costs $12,500 to perform. (It would actually be a lot more, but I want to avoid shocking

PROJECT MAP

1. Think through your research question.
2. Sketch out the analysis.
3. Collect data for your model.
4. Adjust data.
5. Build your model.
6. *Run and test the model.*
7. Conduct sensitivity analysis.
8. Write it up.

anyone reading this book.) We also know that the Reinkenshein procedure costs an additional $10,000 in patent fees to perform, bringing the cost of this procedure up to $22,500. (Look at the initial cost entries in Figure 8.6.)

In Chapter Four, you learned that both costs and effectiveness values must be discounted, and at the same rate. In this case, the cost of the procedure is incurred at birth, so there is no discounting applied. Therefore, we'll want to discount only the HRQL values we enter into these models. (Recall that the Panel of Cost-Effectiveness in Health and Medicine's reference case uses a discount rate of 3 percent.)

Figure 8.7 shows the model with the discounting equation (HRQL/1.03^time) added. Remember that the time that passes is represented as _stage, so the formula is HRQL/1.03^_stage.

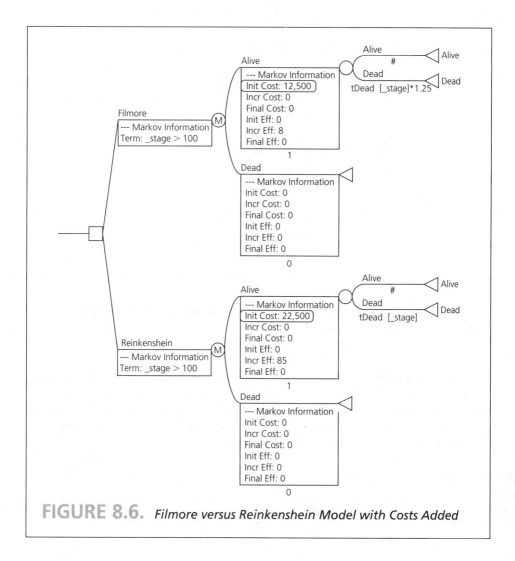

FIGURE 8.6. *Filmore versus Reinkenshein Model with Costs Added*

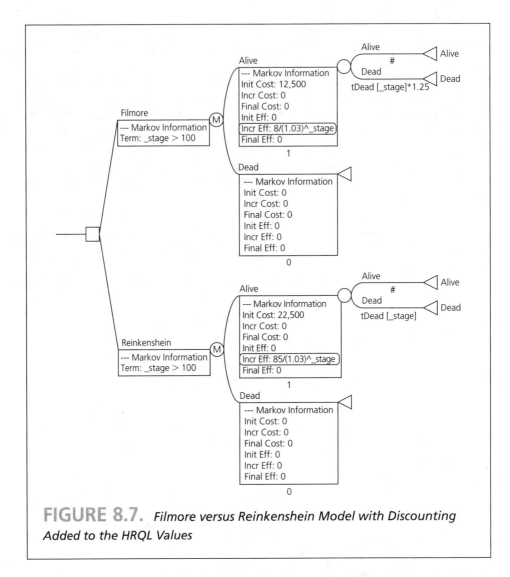

FIGURE 8.7. *Filmore versus Reinkenshein Model with Discounting Added to the HRQL Values*

Finally, Figure 8.8 shows the incremental cost-effectiveness of the Reinkenshein procedure. Notice that the gains in QALE have shrunk considerably after we discounted the values. Nonetheless, the incremental cost charged by greedy Ludviga ($10,000) is more than justified by the gains in QALYs (2 QALYs). The incremental cost effectiveness is just $5,000 per QALY gained.

EXERCISES 5 TO 9

You are running a small needle exchange organization for intravenous drug users in Lagos. You estimate that the program will reduce the seroprevalence of HIV infection by 5 percent among

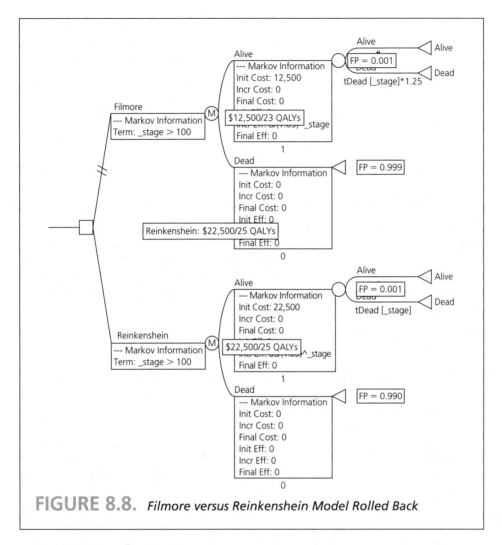

FIGURE 8.8. *Filmore versus Reinkenshein Model Rolled Back*

a group of subjects who are being treated for HIV infection. You look through the literature and are able to find the cost of treating HIV for a year ($1,000). You also know the cost of running the program for one year ($100,000) and life expectancy for HIV-negative persons (20 years) and HIV-positive persons (15 years).

5. You are asked to evaluate the cost returns associated with one year of operation. Which costs are counted over the one-year period, and which costs go beyond this one-year period? (Hint: Think about the future cost savings associated with the initial investment.)

6. You estimate that the program prevents 100 cases of HIV per year. How much money will preventing these 100 cases save over their lifetimes? Assume that none of the cases prevented by your program will later become infected with HIV.

7. What is the lifetime cost savings of the 100 cases in exercise 5 at a 3 percent rate of discount? Recall that the formula is: $Cost/(1.03)^t$, where t is time in the future. For simplicity, assign year 1 savings equal to $1,000 and begin discounting in year 2.

8. HIV-positive patients in Lagos have an average HRQL score of 0.6. What is their discounted quality adjusted life expectancy? (Use a discount rate of 3 percent here too.)

9. HIV-negative persons in Lagos have an average HRQL of 0.9. What is the incremental gain in QALYs per HIV case prevented? (Again, assume that none of the subjects for whom HIV was prevented in year 1 will later become HIV positive.)

DISABILITY-ADJUSTED LIFE YEAR (DALY)

The disability-adjusted life year (DALY) is sometimes used in international cost-effectiveness analyses. Because it was designed for burden-of-disease analysis, it's meant to estimate years of perfect health lost rather than gained. For this reason, the DALY score is equal to 1 − HRQL. Thus, if the HRQL is 0.9, the disability weight is 1 − 0.9 = 0.1. Likewise, to convert a DALY score to an HRQL score, we can simply subtract it from 1.0. The scores have been published in a huge book by Murray and Lopez (1996) and are available for many conditions and diseases.

The general formula for the DALYs lost to disease is:

$$\text{Years of life lost (YLL) + years lost to disability (YLD).} \qquad (8.4)$$

In other words, we first add up the future years of life lost for every death and then add up all of the years of perfect health lost while the individual was still alive to get the total DALYs lost. Thus, if a 30 year old dies who was expected to live to 80, the years of life lost (YLL) is 80 − 30 = 50 DALYs. If those 30 years of life had a DALY value of 0.1, then the person also lost 30 × 0.1 = 3 DALYs. The total DALYs lost is 50 DALYs + 3 DALYs = 53 DALYs.

The DALY is not based on the reference case analysis and for many different reasons does not produce a QALY-compatible HRQL score (Gold, Siegel, Russell, and Weinstein, 1996; Gold and Muennig, 2002). For this reason, it generally should not be used in cost-effectiveness analysis. One exception might be in fieldwork in developing countries where no other HRQL measure is available.

CHAPTER

9

CONDUCTING A
SENSITIVITY ANALYSIS

OVERVIEW

AT VARIOUS points in this book, we have seen how the value of model inputs can be difficult to establish with absolute certainty. For instance, HRQL scores can be obtained from various generic preference-weighted instruments, each producing a slightly different number (Gold and Muennig, 2002). Because these differences arise due to differences in the way the studies are designed, they represent a form of nonrandom error. Most model inputs will be derived from a sample and therefore also contain random error. (For a discussion of random and non-random error, see Chapter Eleven.)

We can usually guess the range of plausible values within which the true value might lie. For instance, looking through the literature, we might see that the HRQL score for the disease we are studying varies by roughly 20 percent when using different instruments. We might also know the standard error in datasets or published values. (Again, if standard error is unfamiliar to you, check out Chapter Eleven before going further.) In this chapter, you will learn how to test the effect of this uncertainty on the output of the decision analysis model.

PROJECT MAP

1. **Think through your research question.**
2. **Sketch out the analysis.**
3. **Collect data for your model.**
4. **Adjust data.**
5. **Build your model.**
6. **Run and test the model.**
7. *Conduct sensitivity analysis.*
8. **Write it up.**

The inputs we are least likely to be certain about are the assumptions we have made. For example, we might have made an assumption about the amount of time it takes for a nurse to administer the influenza vaccine. There are other values that we might be fairly confident about, such as the cost of the influenza vaccine itself. (The average wholesale price is usually easy to get.)

The parameters we are least certain about should be tested over the widest range of values (because it is plausible that the values are much higher or much lower than our baseline estimate). Parameters that we are somewhat more confident about can be tested over a narrower range of values. When a particular strategy remains dominant over the range of plausible values for the inputs that we are uncertain about, the model is said to be **robust**.

There are many different ways of testing variables in a sensitivity analysis. In a **one-way** (univariate) sensitivity analysis, a single variable is tested over its range of plausible values while all other variables are held at a constant value. In a **two-way** (bivariate) sensitivity analysis, two variables are simultaneously tested over their range of plausible values while all others are held constant. In a **multiway sensitivity analysis**, more than two variables are tested. And in a **tornado analysis** (or influence diagram), each variable is sequentially tested in a one-way sensitivity analysis. The tornado analysis is used to rank-order the different variables in order of their overall influence on the magnitude of the model outputs.

Sensitivity analyses can also be used to test for errors in the decision analysis model. By showing how a variable affects the output of a model over a range of values, a sensitivity analysis will bring to light inconsistencies in the model's design. This chapter concludes with a discussion of Monte Carlo analysis, which allows the researcher to generate a confidence interval around the cost-effectiveness ratio.

Because the actual value of any given model input is almost always unknown, we usually enter the inputs as variables in the decision analysis tree rather than a fixed

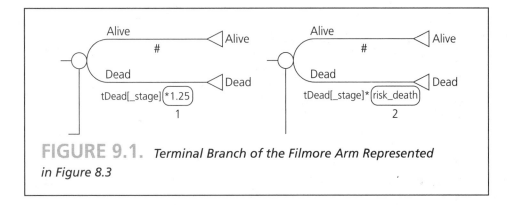

FIGURE 9.1. *Terminal Branch of the Filmore Arm Represented in Figure 8.3*

number. A variable is a kind of placeholder for a number. It can assume a range of values rather than one fixed value. In Chapter Eight, we saw that those who had the Filmore procedure were at 25 percent greater risk of mortality. To measure this higher risk of mortality, we multiplied the annual mortality rate by 1.25. But we might have obtained this 1.25 risk of death from a study that found that the higher risk of death was 1.25 with a 95 percent confidence interval of 1.1 to 1.4. So there is a small chance that the value could be 1.1 and a small chance that the value could be 1.4, but most likely the real-world value is closer to 1.25.

Rather than enter a value of 1.25 here, we can enter a variable (Figure 9.1), which we will call "risk_death." We can now assign risk_death a range of values rather than a fixed number. We can also assign it a **baseline value** so that whenever we roll back the tree, this variable assumes a value of 1.25. The range of values that this variable might assume comes into play only when we conduct a sensitivity analysis on the overall model.

ONE-WAY SENSITIVITY ANALYSIS

What happens to the incremental effectiveness of the Reinkenshein intervention when we vary the effectiveness between 1.1 and 1.4? If we entered each value by hand and then calculated the effectiveness by scratch each time, we might come up with a plot of effectiveness values that looked something like Figure 9.2. This type of analysis is called a one-way sensitivity analysis because we held all other variables constant while changing only the risk ratio of mortality among the recipients of the Filmore procedure.

Here, we see that the greater the risk of death among recipients of the Filmore procedure, the greater the incremental gain in QALYs for recipients of the Reinkenshein procedure. Of course, if the Filmore procedure turns out not to put recipients at increased risk of death, then both procedures will be equally effective.

Just as we can assign variables to effectiveness data, we can assign variables to costs. Let us briefly return to the question of vaccine costs in the influenza research

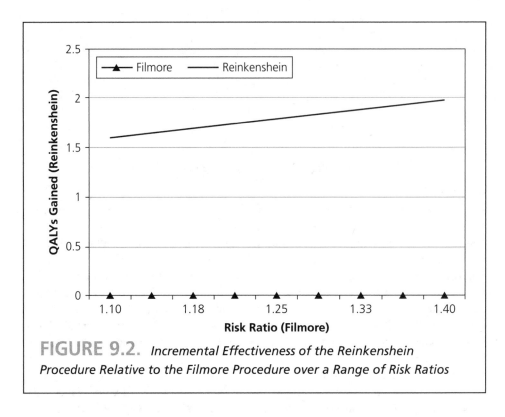

FIGURE 9.2. *Incremental Effectiveness of the Reinkenshein Procedure Relative to the Filmore Procedure over a Range of Risk Ratios*

question. Suppose that we were comparing three strategies: supportive care, vaccination, and treatment with anti-influenza drugs. We want to know the overall cost of each of these strategies when we vary the cost of the vaccine. Now suppose that we're unsure about the cost of providing the vaccine itself, and we think it might vary between $6.99 and $48.79.

In Figure 9.3, the *y*-axis indicates the expected value (overall cost) of each strategy, and the *x*-axis indicates the different vaccine costs at which the model was tested. For example, if the cost of the vaccine were $6.99, the expected cost of the Vaccinate arm of the decision analysis model would be about $32 per person, and the Support arm would cost around $44. The Treat strategy comes in at $49 per person.

Note that the Vaccinate and Support arms cross at $20.92. This means that if the cost of the vaccine were $20.92, the model predicts that the strategy of vaccinating all subjects would cost about the same amount as providing only supportive care. When a variable is set to a value that changes the dominance of one intervention relative to another (the point at which one intervention becomes more cost-effective than another), the value is called the threshold value of that variable.

If the cost of the vaccine were $48.79, our model predicts that the strategy of vaccinating all persons in our cohort would cost around $77—about $28 more than the cost of providing supportive care alone and $7 more than the cost of providing treatment with an anti-influenza drug.

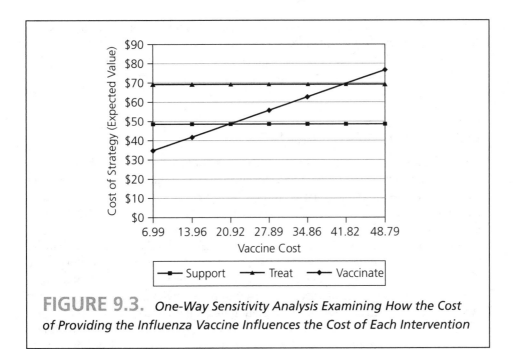

FIGURE 9.3. *One-Way Sensitivity Analysis Examining How the Cost of Providing the Influenza Vaccine Influences the Cost of Each Intervention*

EXERCISE 1

1. Below what cost of the influenza vaccine does the vaccination strategy dominate all other strategies? Above what cost is it dominated by all other strategies?

Using One-Way Sensitivity Analyses to Validate a Model

When examining the results of a one-way sensitivity analysis, always ask yourself whether the expected value of a strategy changes in a predictable way. For example, in Figure 9.3, we would expect that the vaccination strategy would become increasingly less attractive as the cost of the vaccine increases. We would also expect that the amount paid for the influenza vaccine would have no influence on the expected value of any of the other strategies. Thus, they should appear as straight lines (assume the same expected value at all costs of the vaccine).

The easiest way to test that the model has no glaring errors is to consider how you might expect changes in a particular cost or probability to affect a model and then to vary that cost or probability over a wide range of values. Varying a probability from zero to one, or a cost from zero to a very large number, allows you to see the relationship between the strategies under study at predictable end points.

Answering Secondary Questions Using One-Way Sensitivity Analyses

One-way sensitivity analyses are frequently employed to address clinical or policy questions that are not directly related to the primary research question. For instance, we might wish to conduct a broad one-way sensitivity analysis on the cost of oseltamivir, the drug used to treat influenza virus infection. If we demonstrate that there is a price point for this medication that renders it cost-effective relative to the other strategies, the pharmaceutical company that makes the drug may wish to lower its market price.

TWO-WAY SENSITIVITY ANALYSIS

Many variables in a cost-effectiveness analysis are interdependent. For instance, the effectiveness of influenza vaccination is dependent on both the incidence rate of influenza (or the more commonly measured influenza-like illness) and the efficacy of the vaccine in preventing influenza. If the vaccine is 100 percent effective but the incidence of influenza is 0 percent, there is little gain associated with vaccination.

Now suppose that we overestimated the mean efficacy of the influenza vaccine in our hypothetical example. Vaccination might still have been cost saving as long as the overestimation was not large. But if both our estimate of the incidence rate of influenza-like illness and our estimate of vaccine efficacy were too high, the cost savings that we initially found to be associated with vaccination might not be real.

In Figure 9.4, any intersection of values on the x-axis and the y-axis will fall into one of two zones: solid or clear. Each zone indicates which arm will be dominant with

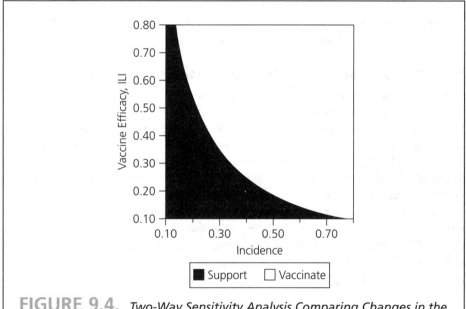

FIGURE 9.4. *Two-Way Sensitivity Analysis Comparing Changes in the Efficacy of the Influenza Vaccine and the Incidence of Influenza-Like Illness*

respect to costs. For example, if the efficacy of the influenza vaccine at preventing influenza-like illness were 0.4 and the incidence rate of influenza-like illness was 40 cases per 100 persons, the vaccination strategy would be dominant with respect to cost (because the intersection of these two values falls in the clear zone). However, if the actual efficacy of the influenza vaccine were 0.3 and the actual average annual incidence rate of influenza was 20 cases per 100 persons, then supportive care would be dominant with respect to cost.

ANALYSIS OF INFLUENCE

Conducting sensitivity analyses may seem like a lot of fun the first few times you do it, but no researcher would want to spend an entire week conducting one-way sensitivity analyses on all of the variables used in the model. If we knew which variables had the most influence on the relative cost (or effectiveness) of each intervention, we could focus on just those variables.

An influence analysis (also known as tornado analysis) is a handy way of determining how much influence each of the variables has on the overall model. These analyses, which produce a graph that assumes the appearance of a tornado, conduct a one-way sensitivity analysis on every variable in the model.

In this type of analysis, each variable is tested independently. Students often assume that the program changes all the variables together over their plausible range of values in a mega-variable slugfest. This is not the case. An influence analysis does nothing more than save the researcher from having to test each variable in separate one-way analyses. The analysis that tests all variables at the same time is known as the **Monte Carlo simulation**.

MONTE CARLO SIMULATION

Imagine that your boss has asked you to come up with sampling error associated with the average cost of hospitalization for influenza infection among a cohort of people infected with influenza in Brazil. The cost was calculated by multiplying the probability of hospitalization by the average cost of hospitalization using a national dataset. You are told that the probability is 0.0002 with a standard deviation of 0.00005 and that the cost is US$500 with a standard deviation of US$50. You know that the average cost of hospitalization among this group is $0.0002 \times US\$500 = \$0.1$, or 10 cents. But what is the standard deviation of this 10-cent value? The problem is that when you have two variables, each with its own standard deviation, it's no simple task to figure out what the standard deviation of the product of these two variables might be.

Now imagine that instead of trying to figure out what the error is for two variables, you must estimate the cumulative effect of the error in 20 variables on your cost-effectiveness model output. Theoretically, if all the variables were associated with sampling error alone, you should be able to estimate a 95 percent confidence interval around your incremental cost-effectiveness value. But how?

One solution is Monte Carlo simulation. Named after the famous gambling enclave, this type of analysis allows the generation of a single confidence interval around multiple variables. In a Monte Carlo simulation, a hypothetical cohort of subjects enters into the decision analysis model. As subjects pass through the model, they encounter a number of different probabilities, such as the chance of developing influenza-like illness, the chance of seeing a doctor, and the chance of being hospitalized. Each time a subject encounters one of these variables, the value that the variable assumes is determined by its probability distribution. (If the word *probability* coupled with the word *distribution* sounds daunting to you, read Chapter Eleven for a quick and simple brush-up on biostatistics. It's easy to understand and will be well worth the time spent.)

For instance, imagine that the cost of hospitalization for influenza in Brazil is US$500 with a standard deviation of US$50, and say that the cost is normally distributed (Figure 9.5). We know that there is a 68 percent chance that the actual cost of hospitalization is between −1 and 1 standard deviations from the mean. When the decision analysis program samples this distribution, it will sample between US$450 and US$550 approximately 68 percent of the time since those values lie within 1 standard deviation of the mean. The chance that a cost will be sampled around 2 standard deviations

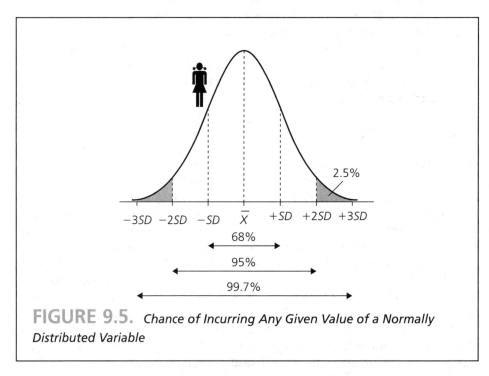

FIGURE 9.5. *Chance of Incurring Any Given Value of a Normally Distributed Variable*

Note: The female figure is at −1 standard deviation from the mean. If the mean is $500 and the standard deviation is $50, this subject would be assigned a value of $450.

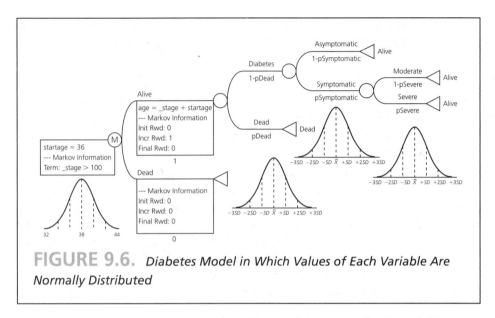

FIGURE 9.6. *Diabetes Model in Which Values of Each Variable Are Normally Distributed*

Note: Each time a subject is run through the model, the subject is assigned a value sampled from each distribution. As a result, the expected value of the variable is normally distributed. In this case, the baseline-expected QALE associated with diabetes is 38 QALYs, but there is a 2.5 percent chance that it could be as low as 32 QALYs or as high as 44 QALYs.

above or below the mean is just 5 percent, with a 2.5 percent chance of a high value and a 2.5 percent chance of a low value.

In a Monte Carlo simulation, the process of running subjects through the model and sampling at each variable is repeated thousands of times. Once the simulation is completed, the expected value of each arm of the decision analysis model will be associated with a distribution of incremental cost or effectiveness values (Figure 9.6).

To look at this in more detail, let's examine the tree that was built to capture the expected value of diabetes in Chapter Seven (see Figure 7.2). Pretend for a moment that all of the variables in this model are normally distributed. At the first juncture, the model samples pDead, it then samples pSymptomatic, and finally, it samples pSevere. If thousands of subjects run through the model, the mean value of each of these variables will determine the expected value of the overall model (38 QALYs). The model now has a distribution of samples as well and can report the approximate 95 percent confidence interval around the mean incremental cost-effectiveness.

Picking Distributions

When the time comes to conduct a Monte Carlo simulation, you may find that few of the variables you wish to include in your model are normally distributed. For example, you may have a series of influenza incidence values you obtained from the medical literature. Even if each study was conducted in a similar way, the mean value in each study will probably resemble the mean value in other studies. This occurs because there is often more than random error involved in generating each mean.

TIPS AND TRICKS

Always be certain to save a backup copy of your decision analysis tree under a different name before you assign distributions to the variables in your model. Once a distribution has been assigned to a variable, you will not be able to conduct further *n*-way sensitivity analyses using fixed probabilities or costs.

For instance, you might be studying the effect of influenza vaccination on the average German, but have data on samples from three different studies in different parts of Germany. Differences in the geographical location of the study and the income, race, and age of the subjects studied can also lead to very different results because the north of Germany is very different from the south. The best way of dealing with this variation is to conduct a meta-analysis. But when a meta-analysis isn't possible, you can pick the value that you think is most likely and a high and low value that you think is quite unlikely, and then artificially distribute your values.

FOR EXAMPLE

Meta-Analysis

In cases in which many similar studies are available, the ideal way to obtain a value for your decision analysis tree is to conduct a meta-analysis and then use the resulting distribution. A meta-analysis provides information about the mean value and a confidence interval from two or more different studies. Meta-analysis is beyond the scope of this book but typically involves selecting many separate studies with a sound research design and then analyzing the data across all studies as if they were a single study. As long as you've been careful in selecting your studies, though, a Monte Carlo simulation comes fairly close to accomplishing what a meta-analysis would without as much effort.

No matter what distribution you use, the final sample will be normally distributed. One preferred way of distributing the values is using a **triangular distribution**. In this distribution, the lowest and highest values are assigned a probability of zero, and the middle value is assigned the highest probability (Figure 9.7). This distribution is unpretentious. It tells the reader that you are unsure what the distribution looks like but that you want low values and high values to be sampled infrequently. You should, however, experiment with different distributions to see how they might influence your model outputs. One great thing about a Monte Carlo simulation is that even if you distribute your values using triangular distributions, the incremental cost-effectiveness value will still be normally distributed!

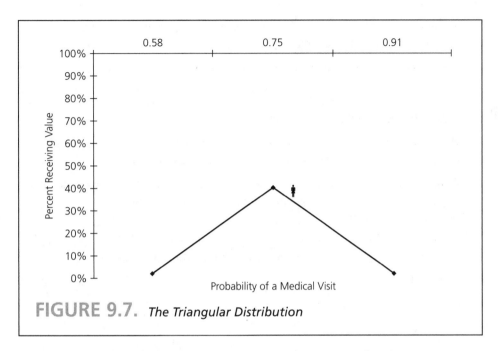

FIGURE 9.7. *The Triangular Distribution*

Note: I have distributed the variable representing the probability of a medical visit using a triangular distribution. The values fall into a range from 0.58 to 0.91, with a middle value of 0.75. The chance of sampling the middle value is 50 percent, but the chance of sampling either extreme is 0 percent.

TIPS AND TRICKS

When a tree containing distributions is rolled back, the average cost or effectiveness values assigned to each arm of the decision analysis model may differ from those generated from a tree that does not contain distributions. This occurs because the mean or midpoint value of the distributions you enter may not be equal to the baseline value you used for each variable.

DETERMINING THE PLAUSIBLE RANGE OF EACH VARIABLE

There are a few guiding principles to follow in determining the range of plausible values for a given variable. These principles can be applied to *n*-way sensitivity analyses and Monte Carlo simulations alike:

- If the parameter is based on an assumption or expert opinion, it should be tested over a very broad range of values in a one-way analysis. Expert opinion should also be used to determine the plausible high and low boundaries for the variable.

- If the parameter was derived from a random sample, you may use 95 percent confidence intervals when most of the error in the value of a parameter will be sampling error. But you should consider ways that nonrandom error may also influence your estimated value.

- If multiple estimates of the value of a parameter are available, consider conducting a meta-analysis or setting the lowest and highest believable values as boundaries in your analysis. You might use these high and low values as end points in a Monte Carlo simulation and opt not to conduct a meta-analysis.

- If two sources of error are interdependent, conduct a two-way sensitivity analysis on each source of error. Do not go overboard with two-way analyses, though!

- If the parameter was obtained from electronic sources, check the data documentation for error estimates. Many data sources comment on both random and nonrandom sources of error.

In addition to some of the principles highlighted here, Gold, Siegel, Russell, and Weinstein (1996) describe methods for conducting more sophisticated sensitivity analyses.

CHAPTER

10

PREPARING YOUR STUDY FOR PUBLICATION

OVERVIEW

THE PUBLICATION format of cost-effectiveness analyses differs from that of other types of scientific investigations in subtle ways. In a cost-effectiveness analysis, the basic format is the same as that of other medical studies; however, the methods and results sections are presented in a way that is structurally quite different from most other studies.

▪ ▪ ▪

CONTENT AND STRUCTURE OF COST-EFFECTIVENESS ARTICLES

Unless the analysis is a **piggyback study** (following a cohort in a prospective study), the description of the cohort is brief, and the first table is often used to describe the values assigned to each variable rather than demographic characteristics, as is done in traditional studies. The second table sometimes includes the assumptions of the study, especially if there are too many to fit easily in the text, but most often contains the incremental cost-effectiveness table.

PROJECT MAP

1. **Think through your research question.**
2. **Sketch out the analysis.**
3. **Collect data for your model.**
4. **Adjust data.**
5. **Build your model.**
6. **Run and test the model.**
7. **Conduct sensitivity analysis.**
8. *Write it up.*

The primary study results are presented using an incremental cost-effectiveness table, which lists the incremental cost and effectiveness of each outcome in ascending order of effectiveness (Gold, Siegel, Russell, and Weinstein, 1996). Outcomes are listed at the standard discount rate of 3 percent (for studies outside the United States, the results should be listed at the prevailing discount rate). The incremental cost-effectiveness ratios should also be presented at various discount rates so that the reader can get a sense of how discounting affects the robustness of the results.

Secondary study results include sensitivity analyses on those variables that are less certain or are central to the analysis. For instance, a cost-effectiveness analysis focusing on interventions for infectious disease in most cases will present a sensitivity analysis on the incidence or prevalence of the disease (Muennig, Pallin, Sell, and Chan, 1999). As in prospective or retrospective studies, the discussion summarizes the findings, discusses the relevance of the findings, discusses the limitations of the study, and makes concluding remarks. Because cost-effectiveness analyses require a good deal of detailed work, it is sometimes necessary to prepare a technical appendix describing the details of your analysis.

In presenting the results of a cost-effectiveness analysis, the researcher has to make a trade-off between the practical and the ideal. Ideally, a cost-effectiveness article will detail every assumption made, outline the entire event pathway, present every formula used, and convey all of the results of the analysis to the reader. In the real world, journal articles are limited to three thousand to five thousand words, so it is important to be concise, and it is often necessary to leave out less critical information. But if too much information is omitted from the journal article, readers will not be able to verify that you have done the hard work necessary to produce a valid cost-effectiveness analysis, let alone replicate it. As with any other study, every cost-effectiveness article contains an introduction, methods, results, and discussion section. In the next few sections, I highlight how these differ from other articles.

INTRODUCTION

The introduction should begin by describing the impact of the disease under study and the need for a cost-effectiveness analysis that evaluates the interventions used to treat or prevent this disease. We will refer to the former as the impact statement and the latter as the statement of need. The impact statement describes the epidemiological and economic impact of a disease on society. The statement of need outlines why there is sufficient uncertainty to warrant the analysis.

The impact of the disease on society usually includes facts pertaining to the incidence rate, the disease severity, or mortality associated with the disease. For example, the influenza article might begin, "Influenza virus infections account for approximately 30,000 deaths, upward of 200,000 hospitalizations, and over a million ambulatory care visits and days of lost work in the United States each year" (Neuzil, Reed, Mitchel, and Griffin, 1999; Nichol, Margolis, Wuorenma, and Von Sternberg, 1994). If the economic impact of the disease has been published elsewhere, these data and their sources might be cited.

When describing the need for a cost-effectiveness analysis, the researcher should indicate why it is unclear whether the costs, risks, and efficacy of one intervention might outweigh those of another. For example, the cost-effectiveness of vaccination versus supportive care hinges on the fact that vaccination must be administered to every healthy adult (Muennig and Khan, 2001). But it's also quite clear that the elderly or chronically ill should be vaccinated since they are at high risk of death or complications if they get the flu.

You might try something like this: "Although there is good evidence that the chronically ill and elderly will benefit from vaccination, healthy adults are at lower risk of hospitalization or death from influenza-virus infections. Nevertheless, complications do arise among younger persons, and otherwise healthy persons can spread disease to the elderly and infirm. Therefore, there is uncertainty as to whether vaccination is cost-effective among healthy adults." Here, you are telling the reader that the analysis will help solve a critical policy question.

A large part of the art of writing journal articles is in the prose. Avoid the use of jargon and painstaking detail. The introduction and discussion sections are less formal and technical than the methods and results sections. Therefore, you should take the opportunity to clearly set up the story you intend to tell in the introduction and tie it all together in the conclusion section.

METHODS

The methods section contains more detailed technical terms; nonetheless, it should be written for the audience of the journal you are submitting to. If it is a journal of epidemiology, use epidemiological terms; most of your readers will have a master's degree or doctorate in this field. If it is a journal geared toward policymakers, consider moving the technical details to the technical appendix.

The methods section should include this information:

- The demographic profile of the cohort or hypothetical cohort

- The perspective of the study (societal, governmental)

- The discount rate used

- The year to which all costs were adjusted

- All assumptions used in the analysis

- Whether the model adhered to the reference case scenario recommended by the Panel on Cost-Effectiveness in Health and Medicine

- The basic event pathway of your analysis

- The sources used to obtain cost and effectiveness data

- The types of sensitivity analyses performed

If you are using a hypothetical cohort, mention how the subjects from your different data sources matched or deviated from your cohort. If differences existed, explain how the problem was addressed.

Details such as the perspective of the analysis, the discount rate used, and the year to which all costs were adjusted can be fit into a single sentence, and the assumptions you used can be put in a table. Placing the assumptions in a table is convenient for a number of reasons. First, one of the nagging difficulties with writing a journal article is that the word count has to be kept within the journal's limits. By placing the assumptions in a table, they are not counted as words in the body text. Second, the reader does not have to scan through the text to find them.

It is important to indicate whether your results include a reference case scenario (or whether the entire study is a reference case analysis). You should also indicate ways in which your results may have strayed from the reference case scenario. For instance, you may not have been able to capture an environmental cost that was likely to have been relevant, or you may not have used a QALY-compatible health-related quality-of-life instrument (Gold, Siegel, Russell, and Weinstein, 1996).

The event pathway should be described in as much detail as possible given the space limitations. Frequently, the decision analysis model will be too large to include in the analysis, and the event pathway will be too detailed to describe. If this is the case, be sure to highlight the key points of the pathway. If you generated the event pathway using clinical practice guidelines, you may wish to cite the guidelines you used.

The bulk of the methods section describes the sources of the cost and effectiveness data you used in your analysis. It should include descriptions of the ways in which you adjusted your data using secondary sources and formulas.

RESULTS

The results section of a cost-effectiveness analysis should include the cost, effectiveness, and incremental cost-effectiveness (if the intervention is not cost saving) of each intervention under study. It should also contain a presentation of the results of the sensitivity analysis.

There is a standard format for presenting the results of cost-effectiveness analyses in table form (see Table 10.1). In a cost-effectiveness table, interventions are ranked in order from the least effective at the top of the table to the most effective at the bottom of the table. The incremental cost-effectiveness ratios are then sequentially calculated from top to bottom (Gold, Siegel, Russell, and Weinstein, 1996). Some decision analysis packages can generate a publication quality cost-effectiveness table for you.

In a cost-effectiveness table, interventions that are dominated (are both less effective and more costly than others) should not contain incremental cost-effectiveness ratios (Gold, Siegel, Russell, and Weinstein, 1996). Instead, the word *dominated* should appear where you would have placed the ratio. The table should be divided into two or three sections listing the results of the analysis at a 3 percent discount rate,

TABLE 10.1. Cost-Effectiveness Table

Row	Intervention	Total Cost	Total Effectiveness	Incremental Cost	Incremental Effectiveness	Incremental Cost-Effectiveness
		A	B	C	D	E
1	Usual care	Cost of usual care	Total QALYs in usual care cohort			
2	Intervention 2	Cost of intervention − savings from intervention	Total QALYs in intervention cohort	A1 − A2	B1 − B2	C2/D2
3	Intervention 3	Cost of intervention − savings from intervention	Total QALYs in intervention cohort	A2 − A3	B2 − B3	C3/D3

Note: Interventions are first ranked by their effectiveness, with least effective interventions listed first. The incremental cost and incremental effectiveness values are then sequentially calculated. Finally, the incremental cost-effectiveness ratios are presented.

undiscounted results, and the results of the analysis at a 5 percent discount rate or higher (Gold, Siegel, Russell, and Weinstein, 1996).

The sensitivity analysis description should outline:

- The variables that exerted the most influence on the model

- How these variables affected the dominance of each strategy

- The results of bivariate analyses (if any are relevant)

- How assumptions affected the model

- The results of a sensitivity analysis on the discount rate

- The results of statistical analyses, such as a Monte Carlo simulation

- Additional analyses of interest to policymakers

Rather than use technical terms such as *tornado analysis*, it is generally better to make descriptive statements. For example, in describing the influence of each variable, you might state, "The incidence of influenza-like illness, the cost of transportation, and the cost of caregiver support exerted the greatest influence over the relative cost and effectiveness of each intervention." You should also describe how each assumption affected the relative dominance of each strategy in one-way sensitivity analyses.

TECHNICAL APPENDIX

It is somewhat more difficult to communicate the results of a cost-effectiveness analysis effectively than it is to present the methods and results of other studies in the health literature. Therefore, extra care must be taken to ensure that all of the relevant issues are addressed while the less important aspects of the analysis are left out. Still, most of the nuances of the cost-effectiveness cannot adequately be described within the word count limitations of most journals.

By including a technical appendix, you will be able to present to the reviewer every assumption, each piece of data used, and all of the mundane details of the sensitivity analyses performed. The reference case recommends that the event pathway in the decision analysis model be described (including changes in the HRQL in each pathway). Some journals may not accept such supplementary materials. In this case, it is generally acceptable to provide the technical document on the Internet, so that all readers can have access to the details of the analysis if they so desire. Your institution's Webmaster or technical folks should help with the task. Many journals offer to post supplementary materials as well.

 ## TIPS AND TRICKS

Most decision analysis programs do not produce publication quality graphs; however, many programs allow the user to export the information used to build a chart into a spreadsheet program such as Excel (Microsoft), a charting program such as SPSS Graph (SPSS), or an illustration program such as Adobe Illustrator (Adobe Systems).

CHAPTER

WORKING WITH DATA

OVERVIEW

ONE OF the ways that cost-effectiveness analysis is fun is that you get to criticize everyone else's hard work. One of the most often used sources of information in cost-effectiveness analysis is the medical literature, and you must be good at tearing it apart to be certain that you are obtaining the highest-quality data possible. Data for cost-effectiveness analyses are also obtained from electronic data sources, expert opinion, the authors of published studies, and in some cases ongoing randomized controlled trials. Although it is not as fun to criticize electronic data as it is to criticize the medical literature, the same basic sources of error are present in both.

To understand data commonly used in cost-effectiveness analysis, you need to know how to work with rates, how to work with distributions, and how to weight means. This chapter provides a basic overview of the epidemiology skills needed for cost-effectiveness analysis in health. The point of this chapter is not to cover any of these topics in detail. Rather, it's here for readers who don't have a degree in biostatistics or epidemiology and need a review of some of the pieces of those disciplines that are most relevant to cost-effectiveness analysis.

■ ■ ■

REVIEW OF RATES

To understand the medical literature and use data in electronic datasets, you should have a basic understanding of rates and know how to calculate them. Rates fall into three broad categories: crude rates, specific rates, and adjusted rates.

A **crude rate** is defined as:

$$\frac{\text{Number of events occurring in a given year}}{\text{Population at risk of event at the mid-point of the year}} \times 10^n \quad (11.1)$$

"Number of events" in the numerator of equation 11.1 refers to the number of diseases, hospitalizations, deaths, and so on that occur in a population of people. The population at risk in the denominator is the population in which an event might conceivably have occurred. For example, if we knew the number of cases of uterine cancer in the United States during 2007, the population at risk would be all females in the United States at the midpoint of 2007.

The multiplier, 10^n, is usually tacked onto the end of a rate to make the rate easier to understand. While it is not easy to grasp the meaning of the mortality rate for stroke, 0.00013, it is easy to grasp the mortality rate of stroke per 100,000 persons: 13 per 100,000 persons. Very common events are usually described per 100 persons (10^2), and very uncommon events, such as death, are usually described per 100,000 persons (10^5).

Crude rates apply to everyone in the population who could have experienced an event and therefore do not account for differences in the characteristics of different groups of people, such as the elderly or the poor. Older people are generally at much greater risk of disease and death than young people, and poor people are generally at much greater risk of disease and death than wealthy people (Muennig and others, 2005). It is critically important that the rates you use are specific to the age, race, gender, and socioeconomic status of your hypothetical cohort.

Age-specific rates refer to the number of events occurring in a particular age group. For instance, the rate of influenza among 20 to 25 year olds is defined as:

$$\frac{\text{Total cases of influenza among persons 20–25 years old}}{\text{Midpoint U.S. population, persons aged 20–25}} \times 10^n \quad (11.2)$$

One of the sad facts of life is that as people get older, the risk of illness and death increases. If we do not carefully account for differences in the rate of disease for each age group, our estimate of the rate of disease may lead to errors in our analysis.

Consider the case of a hypothetical cost-effectiveness analysis cohort and a cohort obtained from a study in the literature, each with 164,000 subjects (see Table 11.1). Suppose that we wish to apply the mortality rates from the study to our cost-effectiveness cohort, but our cohort contains more elderly persons and the study cohort contains more children and adolescents. Multiplying the age-specific mortality rates from the

TABLE 11.1. **Hypothetical Example of Two Populations with Equal Numbers of Subjects and Identical Age-Specific Mortality Rates, But Different Population Distributions by Age**

Row		1	2	3	4	5
			CEA Cohort		Study Cohort	
	Age	Rate	Number of Subjects	Number of Deaths	Number of Subjects	Number of Deaths
1	0–10	0.00010	10,000	1.00	25,300	2.53
2	10–20	0.00015	15,000	2.25	37,060	5.56
3	20–30	0.00023	20,000	4.50	30,250	6.81
4	30–40	0.00045	40,000	18.00	24,200	10.89
5	40–50	0.00090	25,000	22.50	18,150	16.34
6	50–60	0.00270	30,000	81.00	12,100	32.67
7	60–70	0.00810	15,000	121.50	10,890	88.21
8	70+	0.02430	9,000	218.70	6,050	147.02
9	Total		164,000	469.45	164,000	310.01
10	Crude rate • 10^3			2.86		1.89

study in column 1 by the number of subjects in column 2 yields the predicted number of deaths (column 3) among persons of different ages in our hypothetical cohort. In row 9, we see that the total number of subjects in the cost-effectiveness cohort and the study cohort is identical, but the total number of deaths in the cost-effectiveness cohort is higher than the study cohort because there is a larger number of elderly persons subjected to a higher mortality rate.

The crude mortality rate in each cohort is calculated by dividing the total number of deaths by the total number of subjects. For example, the crude mortality rate in the cost-effectiveness cohort is calculated by dividing the value in column 3, row 9 by the value in column 2, row 9. In row 10, we see that the crude mortality rate is also higher in the cost-effectiveness cohort (2.86 deaths per 1,000 subjects) than it is in the study cohort (1.89 deaths per 1,000 subjects).

Adjusted rates (or standardized rates) account for differences in the characteristics of people in two or more populations. While specific rates apply to subgroups within a population, adjusted or standardized rates account for differences in the characteristics of subgroups between two or more populations.

There are two lessons from this section. First, adjusted rates obtained from a study will have been adjusted to some standard population and will therefore usually be useless for your study. The second lesson is that crude rates also almost always are useless. Whenever you conduct a cost-effectiveness analysis, it is necessary to apply age-specific mortality rates to your hypothetical cohort. You will also need to match other demographic characteristics to the characteristics of your hypothetical cohort.

Prevalence Versus Incidence

Prevalence refers to the total number of cases of a disease in society (it is also referred to as **prevalent cases**). The **prevalence ratio** is the total number of prevalent cases divided by the number of people at risk for the disease. The ratio is often erroneously described as prevalence rate. Because it refers to the proportion or percentage of people with a disease rather than the number of cases that develop over a period of time, it is a ratio rather than a rate.

Recall from Chapter One that the incidence refers to the number of new cases over a period of time, usually one year, and that the incidence rate refers to the number of new cases divided by the population at risk of the disease over a defined period of time. In other words, the incidence rate of diabetes in the year 2007 would include only persons who were newly diagnosed with the condition in the year 2007.

Relationship Between Risks and Rates

Rates, such as incidence rates and mortality rates, are usually good estimators of the risk of disease. The risk of disease is defined as:

$$\frac{\text{Number of events over period}}{\text{Population at the beginning of period}} \qquad (11.3)$$

As you can see, the formula for rates, equation 11.1, is very similar to the formula for risk, equation 11.3. Notice that the denominator of equation 11.1 incorporates the midpoint population for the year in which the events occurred as an estimator of the population in which the events can occur, while equation 11.3 includes all subjects over the same period (Jeckel, Elmore, and Katz, 1996).

Suppose that we followed a group of 1,000 people over a year to see how many would develop influenza-like illness. If 410 subjects develop an influenza-like illness, the risk of developing the flu is $410/1,000 = 0.41$. Rates are typically calculated using information from the general population. In the general population, people are constantly moving, dying, and being born. We use the denominator value with the midpoint of the period over which the events were tabulated (the rate) only when we do not have data on a specific cohort of people who have been followed over time (the risk).

So how might the risk and the rate differ in the real world? Imagine that there was a horrible influenza epidemic in February that wiped out 15 percent of the population. If we were to use the midpoint population of that year, we would be underestimating the population in which the events (cases of influenza) actually occurred. Why? Because those who died of influenza would not be counted by the census workers who come around in June. This would result in an overestimation of the risk of influenza, because the denominator would be smaller than it would have been if the true population of persons at risk for influenza had been known.

Technically speaking, any calculation of the risk of influenza, or any other disease that occurs early or late in the year, should be adjusted to better reflect the risk of disease before it is used in a cost-effectiveness analysis. However, for most diseases, the difference between a risk and a rate will not be large. Therefore, a rate can usually be used in a decision analysis model as a substitute for a measure of risk. (The more doubt we have about it, the larger we make the upper and lower bounds of our sensitivity analysis.)

There are four things to consider when deciding whether a rate is a good estimator of risk. First, the period over which the events occur in the rate should be short (one year or less). If the period is long, the greater the chances are that the events in the numerator will fail to mesh with the population in the denominator. Second, if the event is a death, the proportion of the population affected by the event in the rate should be small (less than 3 to 5 percent). If many people die from the event, the population that is susceptible to the event (the denominator) will shrink, resulting in a rate that is larger than the risk. Third, we must consider whether the event occurs once or many times over the period of measurements. Finally, we must be certain that the susceptible population in the denominator of the rate is truly the population at risk of the event. For example, if we knew the total number of influenza cases and were to apply equation 11.1, it would be tempting to divide the total number of cases in each age group by the total population in each age group. However, some people in the general population will have received the influenza vaccine and will not be as susceptible to infection as those who did not.

If we were epidemiologists rather than cost-effectiveness researchers, we might be more interested in the rate of influenza in the general population than the rate of influenza among unvaccinated people, because we would be more concerned with the severity of the epidemic than some abstract notion of risk. However, in cost-effectiveness analysis, we are more interested in knowing the chances of contracting influenza virus infections among unvaccinated and vaccinated people, and we should be careful to include only unvaccinated subjects in the denominator.

TIPS AND TRICKS

Always be careful to remove the constant (10^n) multiplier when using rates in cost-effectiveness analyses. This may seem obvious, but some published rates appear in decimal form despite the 10^n multiplier. For example, the crude mortality rate per 100,000 persons for tuberculosis was 0.1 in 2006 (National Center for Health Statistics, 2005). To obtain the actual mortality rate, this number must be divided by 100,000, yielding a rate of 0.000001.

UNDERSTANDING ERROR

For every measurement, rate, probability, and cost value used in a cost-effectiveness analysis, there exists a true mean value that is applicable to the hypothetical cohort. For example, there is an average risk of developing influenza-like illness in any given year. Unfortunately, only an omniscient being would know what this value is. Being fallible, humans must rely on imperfect scientific methods to estimate the true value of each input into a cost-effectiveness model. The extent to which the measured value of an input is representative of its real value is referred to as the **accuracy** of that measurement. If the value of the input is similar each time that it is measured, it is said to be **reproducible** or **reliable**.

Once you have obtained the articles from the medical literature that you need to conduct your cost-effectiveness analysis, you must determine whether the information you extract from these articles is likely to be accurate. To evaluate the data for accuracy, you will need to have a basic understanding of the common types of error and statistical distributions (such as the normal distribution), and you will need to understand the different ways in which studies are conducted.

The more you read and systematically analyze the methods sections of original research articles, the more comfortable you will become with judging the quality of these articles. Although the basic elements of biostatistics and epidemiology presented in this section will be sufficient as a brief review of error estimation, students who have never had exposure to epidemiology and biostatistics or have never had to critically read the medical literature will require further study.

The most common types of error found in the medical literature are **random error** and **bias**. The extent to which a value is subject to random error is dependent on the size of the sample from which it was derived. Random error is sometimes referred to as sampling error and can be reduced by increasing the size of a statistical sample. We will see examples of how this works in the section "Frequency Distributions and Random Error" later in this chapter.

Bias, or **nonrandom error**, occurs when error affects the data in a systematic way. Consider surveillance data. These data are obtained by asking physicians who see a patient with a communicable disease of public health importance to fill out a card and send it to a local health department. Because only some physicians take the time to fill out the reporting card, reportable diseases are almost always undercounted. This

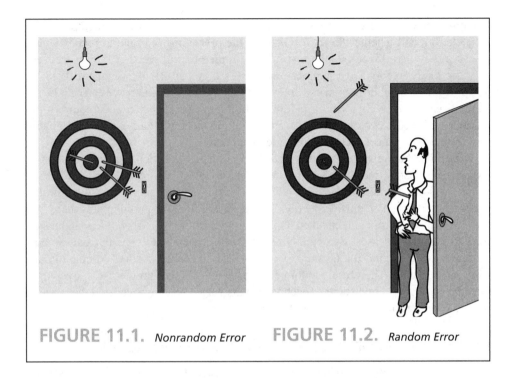

FIGURE 11.1. *Nonrandom Error*   FIGURE 11.2. *Random Error*

type of error is called "nonrandom" because it has nothing to do with the sample size. The error in the number of cases reported always occurs in one direction. Because nonrandom error is systematic, it is sometimes referred to as **systematic bias** or differential error.

To understand the difference between random error and nonrandom error, consider the case of two different people shooting arrows at a target. A highly trained but cross-eyed sharpshooter's target might look like Figure 11.1, while a clear-sighted amateur's target might look like Figure 11.2.

In the first case, the sharpshooter's problem was systematic error or bias. In the second case, the amateur's arrows did not miss the target in a systematic way. Rather, the arrows were randomly distributed around the target. If the amateur kept shooting arrows, the arrows would be distributed around the target in such a fashion that the average distance between arrows was at the center, even if the arrows were scattered all over the wall. Note that this implies that a dataset can be populated with accurate data but contains a good deal of random error. Nonrandom error is, by definition, inaccurate.

Most medical data contain either random or nonrandom error simply because it is very expensive to eliminate both types of error. For example, the National Health Interview Survey (NHIS) is a health survey of about 100,000 people living in the United States (National Center for Health Statistics, 2006a). Because it is administered to a large number of people, it is relatively free of random error when it is used to tabulate the incidence or prevalence of common diseases. However, the NHIS asks subjects to recall whether they were ill over the preceding year and to record which diseases they had. Since people have trouble remembering whether they were sick, they are likely to forget the number of illnesses they had. (If this seems difficult to grasp, try to remember how many times you had a cold over the past year.) Thus, for some diseases, the NHIS will hit below the bull's eye (produce an undercount of the number of diseases respondents had), and it will do so consistently. For unforgettable diseases such as cancer there will be little or no bias.

The NHIS has a sister survey, the National Health and Nutrition Examination Survey (NHANES), that is free of recall bias for most variables; however, the sample size is small (National Center for Health Statistics, 2006b). In this survey, the government parks a huge white van outside the door of unsuspecting citizens and invites them into the van to have their health checked. Once inside, they are poked, prodded, and tested for a number of diseases. By actually testing subjects, the study greatly reduces bias (nonrandom error), but the testing is very expensive, so only a small sample of subjects can be tested. Therefore, random error presents a bigger problem. (To overcome this, the survey is adding subjects each year. This way, researchers can add many years of data together to increase the sample size.)

MANAGING ERROR IN COST-EFFECTIVENESS ANALYSIS

Virtually every source of data you will use in cost-effectiveness research will be subject to random or nonrandom error. Cost-effectiveness researchers must therefore learn how to manage error and demonstrate how error affected the accuracy and reliability of the cost-effectiveness ratios they present to the people who read the analysis.

Random error is usually easy to measure, but nonrandom error cannot always be perfectly quantified. Sometimes, though, it is possible to estimate the extent to which an input is subject to nonrandom error and adjust the input accordingly. This process is akin to nudging the sharpshooter depicted in Figure 11.1 a little to the left. For example, as we learned in the chapter on costs, the amount a hospital charges its clients is known to consistently be an overestimate of the actual cost of providing medical services (Chrischilles and Scholz, 1999). The cost-to-charge ratio is one example of how to reduce systematic bias in your parameter estimate. In other cases, there may be published data on the direction and magnitude of the error. For instance, in self-report surveys, men are likely to overestimate their height, and women are likely to underestimate their weight. Using data from surveys in which a third party measures height and weight, it is possible to obtain a correction (Strauss, 1999).

In many cases, you will not have a good adjuster like a cost-to-charge ratio or a correction from a published study. In such instances, your best hope is to examine the impact this error might have on your incremental cost-effectiveness ratios using a sensitivity analysis. Recall that a sensitivity analysis is a way of testing the effect of error inherent to each input on the overall cost and effectiveness of each of the interventions under study.

Frequency Distributions and Random Error

Suppose we obtain cholesterol test values from 100 people that vary between 115 and 290 mg/dl; the range is 115 to 290 mg/dl. Most of the subjects will have a cholesterol value somewhere close to the mean of these values, but a few will have values around 130, and a few others will have values around 270. If we were to list the number of people who had a cholesterol level between 115 and 135 mg/dl, 135 and 155 mg/dl, and so on, we would have a frequency distribution of these cholesterol levels (see Table 11.2).

If we were to show Table 11.2 graphically, it would take the form presented in Figure 11.3.

The frequency of events can also be described as a probability. For example, the 30 values between 155 mg/dl and 175 mg/dl, out of the 100 subjects in the sample, can be expressed as $30/100 = 0.3$. When frequency distributions are expressed as probabilities, they are known as **probability distributions**. Figure 11.4 shows the data in Table 11.2 as a probability distribution rather than a frequency distribution.

TABLE 11.2. **Frequency Distribution of Hypothetical Cholesterol Values Obtained from 100 Subjects**

Cholesterol Level (mg/dl)	Number of Subjects
115 to 135	3
135 to 155	15
155 to 175	30
175 to 195	25
195 to 215	12
215 to 235	7
235 to 255	5
255 to 275	2
275 +	1
Total	100

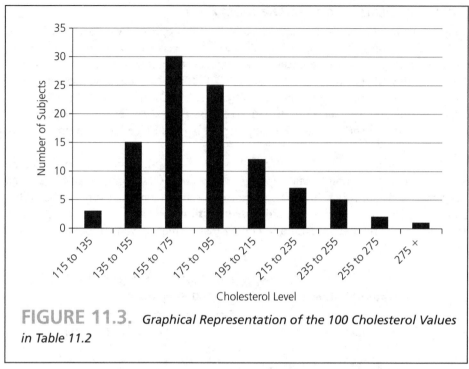

FIGURE 11.3. *Graphical Representation of the 100 Cholesterol Values in Table 11.2*

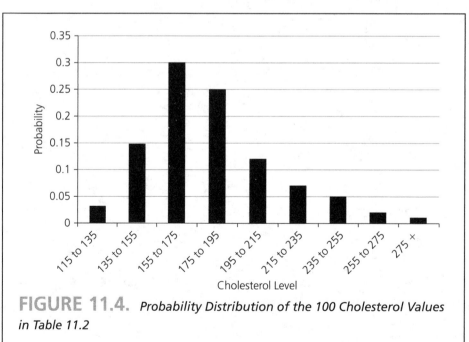

FIGURE 11.4. *Probability Distribution of the 100 Cholesterol Values in Table 11.2*

In Chapter Nine, we saw that the Monte Carlo simulation relies heavily on probability distributions. If we are evaluating a cost-effectiveness analysis of anticholesterol drugs, we will need to incorporate a sensitivity analysis on cholesterol values among untreated subjects. We could simply look at what happens when the mean cholesterol value is 115 mg/dl and when it is 275 mg/dl. But we see from Figure 11.4 that the probability of observing either one of these values is less than 0.05. In our Monte Carlo simulation, we'll want to make sure that values between 155 mg/dl and 175 mg/dl are sampled more frequently than on either extreme. In fact, we'll ideally want these values to come up about 30 percent of the time because that is how often they were observed in our sample. By using probability distributions in our sensitivity analysis, we can ensure that we are commonly observing common values and rarely observing rare values.

Many frequency distributions or probability distributions form a roughly bell-shaped curve known as a **normal distribution** (also known as a *Gaussian distribution*). When perfectly bell-shaped, the peak of the bell (the part that you would hang by a string if it were actually a bell) represents the mean of the sample. When the sample size is small, curves tend to look more like abstract representations of a bell rather than a perfectly drawn bell. (*Skewness* refers to a shift in the peak of a curve to the left or right.) Skewness can occur due to factors other than random error as well, but for now, let's just worry about random error.

If we were to increase the sample size, chances are that more people with high cholesterol levels would be randomly selected, thereby rounding out the curve; as the sample size taken from a normally distributed population increases, the distribution of values looks more and more like an actual bell. If we had a sample size of 1,000 subjects rather than 100 subjects, the probability distribution in Figure 11.4 would probably appear more like Figure 11.5. Thus, as the sample size increases in an unbiased sample of values, the accuracy of the mean value is generally improved.

This brings us to the next point. For any set of numbers, it is, of course, possible to calculate a mean. For instance 1, 2, and 3 have a mean of $(1 + 2 + 3)/3 = 2$. The sum of deviations of these values from the mean is zero. For instance, 1 is -1 units from 2, 2 is zero units from 2, and 3 is $+1$ units from 2. The sum of the deviations is $-1 + 0 + 1 = 0$.

If we were to calculate the average deviation of these numbers from the mean, however, we would take a different approach. The average deviation, more commonly known as the **standard deviation**, is calculated by first squaring the deviation of each data point from the mean. This gets rid of the negative sign. We then calculate the average across all deviations, and then obtain the square root (to undo the square). This average, or "standard," deviation assumes the form:

$$\sqrt{\frac{(x-\bar{x})^2}{n-1}} \qquad\qquad \textbf{(11.4)}$$

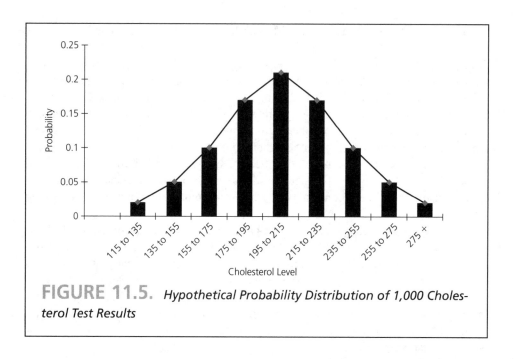

FIGURE 11.5. *Hypothetical Probability Distribution of 1,000 Cholesterol Test Results*

where x is the sample value, $\bar{x}$ is the sample mean, and n is the sample size. (We subtract one from n just to make sure that we are as conservative as possible or "unbiased" in our estimate.) It turns out that if we obtain the standard deviation of any sample, we can know that chance of observing any range of values.

For instance, look at Figure 11.5. The mean of this sample falls at the peak of the curve, or at 205 mg/dl. If the standard deviation of the sample is 30 mg/dl, then cholesterol values between 175 mg/dl and 205 mg/dl fall within 1 standard deviation of the mean. Knowing the standard deviation, we know that values between 175 mg/dl and 205 mg/dl will be observed 34 percent of the time. We also know that anything above or below 30 mg/dl of the mean will be observed 68 percent of the time (see Figure 11.6). The magic of a standard deviation is that it provides us with a uniform probability distribution from which we can infer the chances of observing any one event.

Basics of Statistical Inference

The normal distribution is very helpful for Monte Carlo simulations because it tells us the chance that we will observe any one value. But it has a much more common use in scientific studies.

Studies in the medical literature often compare two or more sample means. For example, a sample of people who are treated with a cholesterol-lowering drug might be compared with a sample of people who are not so treated. If the drug works, the mean cholesterol level in the treated population should be lower than the mean cholesterol level in the untreated population. However, if the sample size is small, differences

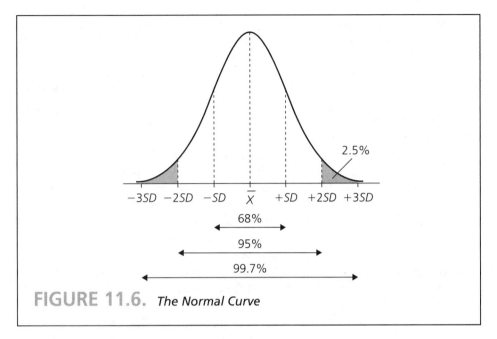

FIGURE 11.6. *The Normal Curve*

Note: SD = standard deviation.

between the two population means must be fairly large for a statistically significant difference to be detected. In other words, if the sample size is too small, it is less likely that a real difference between two population means will be detected. Why? If the sample size is small, the standard deviation will be very large. We will therefore not have a good sense of whether the observed difference is due to random error or a real difference between the mean values. The ability of a statistical test to detect a difference between two population means is referred to as **statistical power**.

In cost-effectiveness analysis, we are interested in knowing the **effect size** of a health intervention. The effect size is the magnitude of the expected improvement realized by an intervention or, more technically, the strength of the measured relationship between two variables. If the observed difference between two means in two small groups is large but the error is also large, we might be overestimating the benefits associated with our intervention.

When a real difference between two populations exists but no difference is detected by statistical testing, it is referred to as a *type II error*. When a difference between two populations is detected by statistical testing but no difference between the means actually exists, it is referred to as a *type I error*.

The possible values of true population means are often presented in the medical literature as measured sample means with 95 percent confidence intervals. The 95 percent confidence intervals refer to the range of possible values of the mean over which we can be 95 percent certain the true value of the parent population mean is represented. In other words, we are saying that any two means that differ by 2 or more standard deviations were probably not observed at random.

Usually researchers are willing to accept a 5 percent probability that the difference between two samples is due to chance alone. When this threshold is set lower, the chance of making a type II error increases and the chance of a type I error decreases. Conversely, when this threshold is set higher, the chance of a type II error decreases and the chance of a type I error increases.

For each variable used in a cost-effectiveness analysis, there is a value that most likely represents the actual cost, probability, or effectiveness measure that we would expect to see in the real world. Recall that this number is sometimes called the baseline value because it will be used to determine the principal cost-effectiveness ratio you will publish in your study. There will also be high and low values for this variable that are plausible (for example, the highest and lowest observed price of a drug on the market).

In cost-effectiveness analysis, researchers will often know that the baseline value is pretty likely and that the high and low values are pretty unlikely, but they will not have any information on the distribution of these values. In these instances, the triangular distribution might be considered (see Figure 11.7).

Let us return to the example of drug costs. Suppose you call ten pharmacies across the country to obtain the cost of oseltamivir. The ten values you obtain might average $53 for a full course of the medication. While the discount drug chains you called were able to sell this medication for less than the mean value, the expensive drug boutique on Rodeo Drive sold it for more. The chance that the actual mean value of this medication is as high as the one you found on Rodeo Drive is very small, and the chance that the mean value is as low as the cheapest drugstore blowout in Joplin, Missouri, is very small. Although you do not have a true statistical sample and do not know the distribution of the values, you want to have a way of telling your decision analysis model that these extreme high and low values are very unlikely. Because you are not certain exactly how unlikely they are, you can simply distribute the probabilities in a triangular shape around the baseline value of $53.

When a triangular distribution is used, values that are more likely representative of the true mean (the baseline values) are assigned a heavier weight than values that represent less likely estimates of the true mean value. In Figure 11.7, the mean cost (about $53 on the left y-axis) is assigned a high probability of occurring (about 0.7 on the right y-axis), based on a subjective assessment of the chance that this is the most likely value for the cost of oseltamivir. Likewise, the extreme low value and extreme high value are subjectively assigned a low probability of occurring.

CALCULATING WEIGHTED MEANS

Weighted means are commonly encountered in cost-effectiveness analysis. Imagine that you had three groups of people randomly selected from the U.S. population to have their blood cholesterol levels measured. Suppose further that you wanted to know the mean cholesterol level of all of the subjects together. If you knew the number of

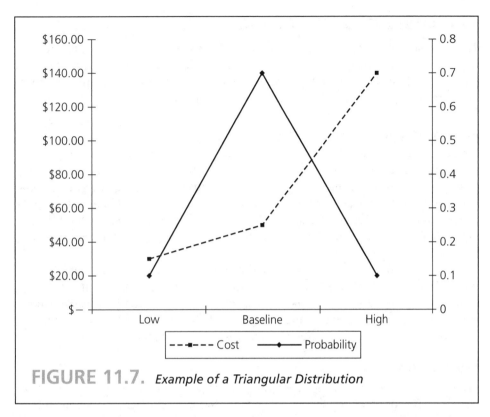

FIGURE 11.7. *Example of a Triangular Distribution*

Note: The solid line represents the probabilistic weight assigned to each cost value represented by the dashed line. Thus, a cost of $140 is assigned a very low probability of occurrence.

people in each group and the mean cholesterol value of each of these groups, you could estimate the overall mean cholesterol level of all of the subjects combined by calculating a weighted mean. A weighted mean is the average value of a set of numbers that are each weighted by some factor, such as the number of subjects in a group.

In cost-effectiveness analysis, it is often necessary to calculate weighted means for the data that you will ultimately use in your cost-effectiveness analysis. If data from many small **cross-sectional studies** are available, a weighted mean can improve the accuracy of a parameter estimate. Means are also useful for adjusting data retrieved from data extraction tools or from printed tabulations of data. A weighted mean is calculated using the formula:

$$\frac{(\text{Events in population 1} \times \text{number of persons in population 1}) + (\text{events in population 2} \times \text{number of persons in population 2})}{(\text{Number of persons in population 1} + \text{number of persons in population 2})} \quad (11.5)$$

EVALUATING STUDY LIMITATIONS

This section explains how to identify limitations of studies and also presents some tips for avoiding research efforts that contain mistakes. However, identifying mistakes on the part of researchers is tricky (and sometimes impossible) given the limited amount of information published in the methods section of a research paper.

Review of Medical Study Designs

Medical studies are usually conducted to evaluate risks or rates. For example, they might indicate the risks associated with smoking or the risk of morbidity or mortality among people treated with a new medication relative to untreated people. Alternatively, they might indicate the probability that a screening test will correctly identify people who have a disease. Because cost-effectiveness analyses are constructed using the probabilities of different events, virtually all cost-effectiveness analyses will require information from medical studies.

Medical studies are usually described according to how they follow subjects over time. While cross-sectional studies give a slice of information at one point in time, retrospective studies examine factors that occurred in the past, and prospective studies are designed to examine events that will occur in the future. Each of these different study designs has different limitations, and it is important to understand them.

Cross-Sectional Studies

In a cross-sectional study, data are obtained at one point in time. Cross-sectional studies are useful for obtaining the prevalence of disease or enumerating the number of people at risk for a particular disease (for example, identifying the number of smokers

FOR EXAMPLE

Placebo-Controlled Studies

The placebo effect is a powerful biopsychological phenomenon. People who are given dummy pills or sham surgery often experience improved health outcomes relative to those that do not. For example, when coronary artery bypass surgery was first evaluated, subjects with angina (chest pain) who were randomized to the placebo group were given nothing more than a superficial cut on the skin of their chest. (Today, this practice would probably not be deemed ethical.) Subjects in the experimental group underwent open-heart surgery. While 70 percent of the patients who received the surgery reported improvement in chest pain, all of the patients in the placebo group reported improvement (Fisher, 2000).

in different age groups). Simple cross-sectional studies can be conducted rapidly using national datasets. For instance, in the United States, the Behavior Risk Factor Surveillance System can be used to determine the percentage of adults who are vaccinated against the influenza virus, the number of smokers, or the number of people with other risk factors for disease.

Retrospective Studies

Retrospective studies are generally designed to identify risk factors for disease. In a retrospective study, people with a disease are paired up with a control group of people who are similar in most ways but do not have the disease. Each group is then examined for a past exposure to some risk factor for the disease (see Figure 11.8). For example, a group of new mothers whose children had cleft palate might be asked about a potential contributing cause, such as having taken a medication while pregnant. A group of mothers whose children were free of birth defects and gave birth in the same hospital might then be interviewed to determine whether they too had taken that particular medication during pregnancy.

Retrospective studies are especially susceptible to bias. For instance, recall bias occurs when the group without the disease fails to remember whether they were exposed to the risk factor. In the case of the new mothers, those whose children had a birth defect may be much more motivated to try to remember whether they had taken medications during pregnancy than mothers whose children did not have the birth defect. If the subjects in the control did not remember having taken the medication (and thus underreport its use), the medication may be falsely implicated as a cause of the birth defect.

Another common type of bias specific to retrospective studies is confounding. This occurs when the control group does not match the experimental group with respect to another risk factor for the disease. For example, one study examining the relationship between coffee drinking and heart disease found a strong association. However, because coffee drinkers are also significantly more likely to smoke than people who do not drink coffee, the control group contained fewer smokers than the experimental group (Thelle, Arnesen, and Forde, 1983; Urgert and others, 1996). (Coffee subsequently was found to be relatively safe.) Because of the great potential for confounding, data from retrospective studies are rarely used in cost-effectiveness analysis.

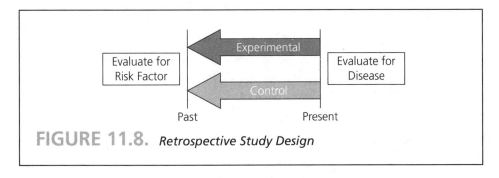

FIGURE 11.8. *Retrospective Study Design*

Prospective Studies

Like retrospective trials, **prospective studies** are generally designed to identify risk factors for disease. Prospective trials offer a number of advantages over retrospective trials. First, they reduce bias by examining people with a putative risk factor relative to those without the potential risk factor before they develop disease. Subjects are then followed over time to see whether the people with the risk factor are more likely to develop the disease (Figure 11.9). Second, they allow the calculation of incidence rates and **risk ratios**. A risk ratio indicates how much more likely people with the risk factor are to develop disease than those who do not have the risk factor.

The risk ratio is calculated as the **incidence rate** of disease among people with the risk factor over the incidence rate of disease in people without the risk factor, or:

$$\text{Risk ratio} = \text{Incidence}_{\text{Risk factor}}/\text{Incidence}_{\text{No risk factor}} \qquad (11.6)$$

which is often written as:

$$\text{Risk}_{\text{Risk factor}}/\text{Risk}_{\text{No risk factor}} \qquad (11.7)$$

The risk ratio is also referred to as **relative risk**. (Both are conveniently abbreviated RR.)

TIPS AND TRICKS

Technically, equation 11.6 refers to a rate ratio rather than a risk ratio. *Risk ratio* is sometimes used when it is important to distinguish between a ratio of rates and a ratio of risks. In practice, these terms are often used interchangeably. (See "Review of Rates" previously in this chapter.)

The risk ratio produces a number that is easy for most people to understand. For example, the relative risk of developing lung cancer among smokers is about 9.0, indicating that smokers are at nine times the risk of developing lung cancer as nonsmokers

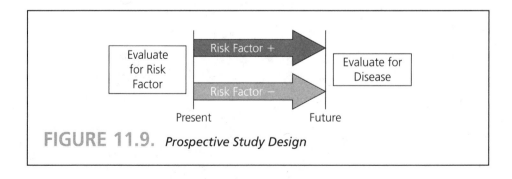

FIGURE 11.9. *Prospective Study Design*

(Doll and Hill, 1956). Retrospective trials allow for the calculation of **odds ratios** rather than risk ratios, a measure that reflects risk only when applied to relatively rare conditions.

Prospective studies are expensive to conduct and are therefore often generally applied only to major research questions relating to common diseases. Older prospective trials were often targeted toward white male cohorts, and the results may not always be generalizable to other populations.

Another problem with prospective studies is that subjects who are willing to participate in a study may differ from those unwilling to participate. People who are willing to take part in a randomized controlled trial without reimbursement may be healthier, more ideological, or more affluent than people who do not, which can distort the overall severity or impact of a disease. For instance, imagine a study that examines the overall impact of smoking on health outcomes. If mostly healthy subjects enroll in the study, people with diabetes might be excluded from both the experimental and control groups. Because a diabetic who smokes is at much greater risk of heart disease than the cumulative risk of both of these conditions separately, smoking may appear to be less harmful than it really is.

The tendency for volunteer study subjects to be healthier than the general population is called the **healthy volunteer effect**. If we were to evaluate a nonsmoking intervention in a cost-effectiveness analysis using data obtained from a cohort of mostly healthy smokers, the benefits of smoking cessation would be artificially reduced.

People who drop out of studies differ from those who stick with a study to the end. For example, in a famous prospective study of risk factors for heart disease conducted in Framingham, Massachusetts, subjects who dropped out of the investigation were later found to have a much greater risk of heart attack and death than the subjects who stayed in the study (Dawber, Kannel, and Lyell, 1951). Prospective studies are commonly referred to as **longitudinal studies**, because patients are followed over time.

Like retrospective studies, prospective studies can be confounded. For instance, people who drink coffee are more likely to smoke. Even if you follow coffee drinkers who are free of heart disease over time, they will still be thought to develop heart disease at a higher rate than noncoffee drinkers simply because they smoke. Therefore, it is important to think long and hard about how the relationship between the risk factor and the disease might be confounded and then ask yourself whether the authors took this into account by controlling for the relevant confounders.

Why so much attention to the problems associated with prospective studies when retrospective studies are so much more problematic? Because they are commonly used as inputs to cost-effectiveness analyses. Therefore, it's very important to understand their limitations.

Randomized Controlled Trials

The **randomized controlled trial** is probably the most often used source of information in the field of cost-effectiveness analysis. A randomized controlled trial is a type of prospective study designed to determine whether those who receive a particular

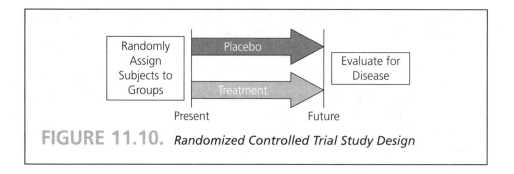

FIGURE 11.10. *Randomized Controlled Trial Study Design*

intervention have better health outcomes than those who do not. In this design, subjects are randomly assigned to either an intervention group or a placebo group (Figure 11.10). They are then followed over time to see if there are differences in the rate or severity of disease between the two groups. The difference between a randomized controlled trial and other prospective studies is that some subjects in other prospective studies have something (such as a smoking problem) that may increase their risk of disease, and some subjects in a randomized controlled trial are given something (such as smoking cessation advice) that may reduce their risk of disease.

In a randomized controlled trial, it is common to control for the placebo effect (see the "For Example" box earlier in the chapter on this topic). Unfortunately, in the field of cost-effectiveness analysis, we are interested in how interventions work in the real world. In the real world, people who take a medication benefit from both the treatment effect and the placebo effect.

When a medical intervention is compared with a placebo and the placebo has an impact on the illness under study, the cost-effectiveness of an intervention will be underestimated. Consider the case of clinical evaluations for minoxidil solution, a topical treatment for male pattern baldness. Balding men do not usually spontaneously grow hair. However, this is exactly what happened with men in the placebo group of some of the randomized controlled trials evaluating the clinical efficacy of this drug (Clissold and Heel, 1987). If we were to measure the effectiveness of the drug relative to the placebo, the drug would appear to be less effective than if it were measured relative to each subject's hair pattern when the study was started.

Other subconscious cues, such as the body language of a researcher, can also have an impact on treatment outcomes in a randomized controlled trial. For this reason, the researchers who actually interact with patients are often made unaware of whether the patient has received the intervention. When neither the patients nor the researchers who interact with the patients know who received the placebo and who received the treatment, the study is said to be **double-blinded**.

To keep both the patients and the researchers unaware of who is in the experimental group and who is in the placebo group, patients must be randomly assigned to either group. The status of each patient is hidden until the end of the study, at which point the study is "uncovered," and the effects of the intervention are examined. It is therefore important to examine the characteristics of the patients who were randomly allocated to the placebo group or the control group (these characteristics are almost always presented in the first table in the article describing the study).

Sometimes chance works against researchers, and subjects receiving the placebo have a lower average income or smoke more often than subjects in the intervention group. When the subjects in the placebo group happen to have more risk factors for disease than the subjects in the experimental group, or imperfections in the randomization process occur, the intervention may appear to be more or less effective than it would have been under perfect conditions. For these reasons, it is important to make sure that the experimental and control groups used in the study are demographically similar. If they differ slightly, the effect size may be more precisely estimated by adjusting for demographic differences between groups.

Meta-Analysis

A **meta-analysis** is a systematic analysis of many studies published in the medical literature. In this design, data are obtained from different prospective or randomized controlled trials and then combined into a single study. For example, if one study evaluated a treatment for heart disease in Chicago and another study evaluated the same treatment using a similar study design in San Francisco, the subjects in the experimental group from each study would be combined into a single group. Similarly, the subjects from the control groups would be combined into a single group. The effect of the treatment on the combined experimental group relative to the combined control group would then be analyzed.

As with any other study, the quality of meta-analysis studies is variable. One recent meta-analysis in a major peer-reviewed journal found that mammography was not effective at reducing mortality rates for breast cancer (Gotzshe and Olsen, 2000). However, the authors chose to exclude all of the studies demonstrating the clinical effectiveness of this technique because they felt that these studies had problems with the random allocation of subjects. Most experts agree, however, that mammography is effective because the mortality rate for breast cancer has declined more rapidly than improvements in treatments would suggest.

When many studies exist pertaining to a particular parameter of interest in a cost-effectiveness analysis, cost-effectiveness researchers sometimes conduct their own meta-analysis on these studies. For example, if it were necessary to generate an estimate of the incidence rate of influenza infection for the United States but only regional estimates were available, a meta-analysis of all of these studies might provide a better estimate of the rate of influenza nationwide. Meta-analytical techniques are too advanced for an introductory textbook, and we encourage you to study the topic in more depth.

Primary Cost-Effectiveness Studies

In some instances, a longitudinal study will be primarily directed at collecting cost and effectiveness data. In this study design, a group of subjects are administered a standard of care intervention and one or more health interventions with the primary goal of determining the cost-effectiveness of a particular strategy. In other words, subjects are allowed to behave as they might in a real-world setting and costs are measured as they are incurred. For instance, if the study were evaluating a new antibiotic, patients may see the physician as they normally do. The time spent during the medical encounter is measured, the cost of the antibiotics is recorded, and no unusual measures are taken to ensure that the patients have taken all of their medications. If patients have side effects to the medication, the researchers determine whether the side effects led to additional medical visits or other costs. Finally, the time patients spend receiving care, driving, and other costs is recorded.

The advantage of a primary cost-effectiveness analysis is that most sources of error can be carefully controlled, costs can be obtained directly from the study, and cost-effectiveness analyses can simulate real-world conditions better than standard longitudinal analyses, providing effectiveness data as well as efficacy data. Unfortunately, try as the researchers may, this approach still yields results obtained under experimental rather than real-world conditions. For instance, patients might be followed in university hospitals where medical care differs from that in other clinical settings. In a traditional cost-effectiveness analysis (an analysis that uses secondary sources of data), it is often possible to examine longitudinal studies from many different parts of the country and in different clinical settings, improving the validity of the analysis.

Generalizability

When evaluating the medical literature, two questions should immediately come to the cost-effectiveness researcher's mind. The first is, "Was this study carefully designed and executed?" The second is, "Are the results of this study generalizable to my study population?" If these two questions are consistently asked, cost-effectiveness researchers should be able to get a better idea of whether the data that they wish to extract from the study will be useful. Although there are a number of good books available for evaluating study quality, most pay less attention to issues of generalizability, which is an issue that is paramount in cost-effectiveness analysis.

Are the results generalizable to your study population? A study with external validity will produce results that are generalizable to groups other than those under study. One criticism of medical research conducted in the twentieth century is that the majority of studies examined only the health effects of white men, raising questions as to whether the study results were valid for other groups in the United States. It may be the case that one type of antihypertensive medication is better for African American males and another is better for white women, but these differences in treatment response are usually not known because those cohorts were not represented in the studies. Sometimes the results of studies are undergeneralized as well. Until recently, women with crushing chest pain were sometimes sent home from the emergency room because heart disease was thought of as a "male problem."

Studies applied to specific subgroups of a population can be especially problematic for cost-effectiveness researchers. For example, a cost-effectiveness analysis examining screening mammography versus no screening among African American females would require tricky assumptions on the part of researchers; most studies of the effectiveness of screening and the effectiveness of various treatments were conducted on cohorts of mostly white women.

The following subsets of questions should help you determine whether the results of a published study are generalizable to your study population:

- *Was the study population localized to a particular geographical region?* Results of studies conducted in a specific geographical region of the country may not apply to all persons nationwide. For example, the rate of influenza-like illness in a study conducted in New York City (where winters are cold and people are packed into subways) may not apply to persons living in Los Angeles (where the weather is nice and people spend most of their time alone in cars). It would be best to obtain a national estimate of influenza-like illness or estimates from other parts of the country for comparison.

- *Are the characteristics of the subjects in the study similar to the characteristics of the population you are studying*? Often, researchers conduct studies in specific settings such as a Veterans Affairs hospital or in a health maintenance organization. In the former case, the patients may be likely to be older and have many coexisting illnesses. In the latter case, the subjects may be more likely to be employed and middle or upper middle class than the general population.

- *What were the inclusion and exclusion criteria?* Sometimes studies examining a treatment for a disease will exclude people with preexisting medical conditions. For example, studies on the efficacy of the influenza vaccine almost always exclude subjects who have diseases that put them at high risk of hospitalization or death from influenza virus infections. Subjects with chronic diseases are excluded from vaccine efficacy studies because subjects in the placebo group have a moderate risk of death if they actually contract influenza. Since we are interested only in the efficacy of the vaccine in healthy adults, this research will be useful to us. However, if we were interested in the efficacy of the vaccine in all adults, the results of these studies would be of little use, because an important subset of our hypothetical cohort would have been excluded (Advisory Committee on Immunization Practices, 2004).

- *Does the definition of illness differ in any meaningful way from the definition you are using, or does it differ from the definition used in other studies you are including in your analysis?* Differences in the way that illness is defined can lead to differences across model inputs. For instance, influenza-like illness can be defined as with or without a fever. Cases containing a fever are much more likely to actually be influenza and are more likely to be severe (de Andrade and others, 2000). If you use a study that doesn't include fever among the complex of symptoms defining the illness to obtain the likelihood of a medical visit, you are likely to underestimate this probability.

■ *Did the subjects who failed to complete the study differ from subjects who successfully completed the study?* Often subjects who drop out of a study or subjects who fail to complete surveys are sicker than the general population or at higher risk of disease. If a large number of subjects failed to complete a prospective study, the risk ratio for the factor under study is likely to be larger in the real world than in the study. As a very general rule of thumb, at least 80 percent of the subjects should complete the study. However, if 100 percent of the subjects in the group without the risk factor under study completed a prospective study and 80 percent of the subjects with the risk factor completed the study, we can expect the results to be skewed. Often researchers look back at noncompleters to make sure that they aren't that different from completers.

■ *How did the treatment and placebo groups differ in demographic composition and risk factors for disease?* In an economic analysis of influenza vaccination (Bridges and others, 2000), a significantly higher number of subjects exposed to second-hand smoke at home were randomly assigned to receive the influenza vaccine than subjects who were randomly assigned to receive the placebo injection in one part of the study. In that season, the influenza vaccine was poorly matched to the circulating strains of influenza virus, and the subjects who received the vaccine had higher rates of influenza-like illness and more medical visits than subjects in the placebo group.

Other Ways of Identifying Error in the Medical Literature

It is standard practice for authors to discuss the limitations of their studies in the discussion section of their research articles. Here, you often find a good deal of qualified language surrounding the major problems with the analysis. In some cases, authors provide in-depth discussions of the problems they encountered with their research. If an editorial accompanies the article, it may identify additional problems with the research. A final forum for identifying problems with a study is to read the letters to the editor in the months following the study. Medline searches help identify the volume and issue in which the letters were published.

CHAPTER

12

FINDING THE DATA YOU NEED

OVERVIEW

COST-EFFECTIVENESS STUDIES often synthesize information from a number of different sources. Usually researchers require information on the incidence or prevalence of a disease, risk ratios, and costs, among many other inputs. These inputs can be obtained from the medical literature, electronic datasets, unpublished sources (such as ongoing longitudinal studies), or experts on the disease you are studying. In this chapter, we examine different sources of publicly available electronic data, briefly discuss the ways in which alternative data sources can be used, and forward a system for organizing the data you collect.

One question that might immediately come to you is, Why is this chapter near the end of the book? As you went through sample cost-effectiveness analyses, you learned about many of the data sources mentioned in this chapter. For example, you obtained hospital costs from the Healthcare Cost and Utilization Survey in Chapter Four. This chapter isn't really meant for students in a cost-effectiveness class. It's meant for those who are hunkering down to conduct their own analysis and need to know where to look for specific types of data.

■ ■ ■

FINDING DATA IN THE MEDICAL LITERATURE

It is generally easy to find the medical literature that you will need for your cost-effectiveness analysis. PubMed is a popular and comprehensive search engine for scientific research that is run by the government and can be accessed on the Internet at http://www.ncbi.nlm.nih.gov/entrez/query.fcgi, which has a helpful tutorial.

GRADING PUBLISHED DATA

In Chapter Eleven, we reviewed some of the basic biostatistics and epidemiology concepts pertinent to cost-effectiveness analysis. That section was intended for those who don't have a degree in one of those two disciplines. If you've read that chapter or are familiar with these concepts, you should have some idea about how research studies are designed and some of the common limitations. But how do you decide which ones to use and which to reject? One approach to evaluating the quality of the published data you have gathered for your cost-effectiveness research project is to apply the **levels of evidence** criteria. Levels of evidence is a grading method for organizing published data based on their trustworthiness (Canadian Task Force, 1979).

One useful way of thinking about the levels of evidence is to visualize it as a pyramid, with the most trustworthy study designs at the top and the least trustworthy at the bottom. Multicenter randomized controlled trials and meta-analysis of these studies cap off the pyramid. Single-site randomized controlled trials make up the next level, evidence from nonrandomized trials the next, and on down to expert opinion.

While grading scientific studies is beyond the scope of an introductory textbook, there are some excellent sources of information available to curious students. An up-to-date discussion of levels of evidence can be found at the Oxford Center for Evidence-Based Medicine (http://www.cebm.net/levels_of_evidence.asp).

Unlike studies in the medical literature, it is relatively easy to identify error in an electronic dataset; most datasets are accompanied by detailed descriptions of the limitations of the data they contain.

USING ELECTRONIC DATASETS

Health datasets provide a wealth of information for conducting cost-effectiveness analyses. Using these datasets, you can obtain much of the information on medical costs, disease prevalence rates, hospital discharge rates, or just about any type of cross-sectional health-related data in which you are interested. Some prospective data are also available. Nonhealth datasets contain information related to transportation, crime, and education, all of which are useful for estimating the nonmedical costs of medical interventions or diseases.

Although the words *electronic* and *dataset* instill a sense of fear in many people, obtaining data from electronic databases is not difficult. In fact, there are a number of tools designed specifically to make the information that electronic datasets contain more accessible to nontechnical types. These tools take the form of computer programs or Web pages that guide would-be researchers through the step-by-step process of obtaining the information they need. These programs or Web pages are sometimes referred to as **data extraction tools**. (In Chapter Four, you used one of these tools to get hospitalization costs from the Healthcare Cost and Utilization Project.)

It is also possible to obtain cost-effectiveness data inputs using printed tabulations of data from these datasets. These are large documents containing lists of useful data, such as hospitalization rates or mortality rates, as well as the most commonly used cross-tabulations. A cross-tabulation lists the outcome of interest (such as a hospitalization rate) by some other characteristic (such as gender).

Virtually all major health datasets in the United States are either associated with a data extraction tool or are available as a printed tabulation (see Exhibit 12.1). The majority of international data sources require familiarity with statistical packages (see Exhibit 12.2). However, the World Health Organization has organized many data sources from developing countries in various user-friendly ways. We assume that those who can use statistical software packages are already familiar with how to find and download the health data they need. If you fall into this category but need guidance, Exhibit 12.1 should get you where you need to go.

EXHIBIT 12.1. Major U.S. Health DataSets Available to the Public

Dataset	Description
Healthcare Cost and Utilization Project-3 (HCUP-3) www.ahrq.gov	This dataset contains information on hospital discharges from 17 states. Data may be obtained for specific states or weighted for national averages. Contains information on the number of discharges by disease, and hospital charges.
National Hospital Discharge Survey (NHDS) www.cdc.gov/nchs	A smaller sample of hospitals than the HCUP-3. This dataset is available in electronic and published form.
Medical Expenditure Panel Survey (MEPS) www.meps.ahrq.gov	Contains survey data from clinicians, nursing homes, and the general population regarding health care use, expenditures, insurance status, and many other useful variables. Useful for generating ambulatory care costs.
National Ambulatory Medical Care Survey (NAMCS) www.cdc.gov/nchs	This is a national survey of physicians that includes over 36,000 patient records for ambulatory care services. Does not include hospital outpatient or emergency room data.

(Continued)

Dataset	Description
National Hospital Ambulatory Medical Care Survey (NHAMCS) ⚙ www.cdc.gov/nchs	This dataset supplements the NAMCS with hospital and emergency room data.
National Nursing Home Survey (NNHS) www.cdc.gov/nchs	This dataset provides information about 8,000 randomly selected nursing home patients.
National Home and Hospice Care Survey (NHHCS) www.cdc.gov/nchs	This is a national sample of 1,500 home and hospice care agencies.
Surveillance, Epidemiology, and End Results System (SEER) ⚙ http://seer.cancer.gov/	This dataset contains information on most major cancers. Variables specific to race, gender, country of birth are linked to census data.
National Health and Nutrition Examination Survey (NHANES). ⚙ www.cdc.gov/nchs	This nationally representative dataset contains data from physical examinations and clinical and laboratory tests. Prevalence data are available for specific diseases and health conditions.
National Health Interview Survey (NHIS) ⚙ 📄 www.cdc.gov/nchs	A nationally representative survey of the health status, mobility limitations, and disease for non-institutionalized persons. Also contains the total number of medical visits for each subject.
Mortality Statistics www.cdc.gov/nchs 📄	Death certificates contain information on all deaths by ICD-9 code and include the decedent's place of birth, education level, location of the death, as well as the underlying cause of death and other conditions the decedent had. These data are contained in a wide array of data formats.
Combined Health Information Database http://chid.nih.gov	Contains a number of datasets related to chronic disease.
Bureau of Labor Statistics www.bls.gov ⚙	Government agency that tracks wages for many professions. This is useful in estimating time costs for patients who undergo an intervention.

⚙ Indicates that a data extraction tool is available. 📄 Indicates that printed tabulation is available.

EXHIBIT 12.2. Major Sources of International Health Data

WHO Statistical Information System, http://www.who.int/whosis/en/

CHOosing Interventions That Are Cost Effective (WHO-CHOICE), http://www.who.int/choice/en/

Unit Costs for Health Services by Country (WHO), http://www.who.int/choice/country/en/index.html

Harvard International Health Data, http://hcl.harvard.edu/research/guides/health_international/

Centers for Disease Control and Prevention, International Health Data Reference Guide, http://www.cdc.gov/nchs/data/misc/ihdrg2003.pdf

OECD Health Data 2007: Statistics and Indicators (provides limited public access data), http://www.oecd.org/

United Nations Statistics Division, http://unstats.un.org/unsd/demographic/products/socind/health.htm

U.S. Department of Health and Human Services: Global Health, http://www.globalhealth.gov/

The advantage of working with an entire dataset is that you will have more control over the ways in which different pieces of information are combined, making it possible to conduct more sophisticated analyses. Because this is an introductory textbook, we will focus on obtaining data from sources that do not require the use of a statistical software package.

TIPS AND TRICKS

Active links to major sources of data useful for cost-effectiveness analysis are maintained at http://www.pceo.org/datasources.html.

Analyses conducted in developing countries previously had to rely on the medical literature or ongoing prospective trials. However, the World Health Organization (WHO) now maintains a useful data repository with information specific to cost-effectiveness analysis (http://www.who.int/choice/en/). In the following sections, we discuss how you can obtain printed data tabulations and data from ongoing studies and how to estimate an input using expert opinion.

Finding the Right Electronic Data

Though electronic datasets are rich sources of information, you will have to familiarize yourself with the contents and limitations of each of the datasets commonly used in cost-effectiveness analysis in your country. Once you are pointed in the right direction, though, it is relatively easy to find the information that you are looking for. For instance, Statistics Canada contains most of the important national health and demographic statistics for Canada (http://www.statcan.ca/start.html). By contacting Statistics Canada officials, it is often possible to find other sources of data, such as provincial health plan datasets that they do not maintain. The same goes for many other countries as well. (See, for instance, http://www.destatis.de/, which contains statistics for most German agencies.) In fact, researchers examining other contexts can often find statistics for European nations in English. (See, for instance, http://www. destatis. de/e_home.htm.)

Most health datasets are designed to meet a particular research need. Therefore, datasets tend to have themes, much the same way that a novel will have a central protagonist and plot. Like novels, some datasets essentially replicate the themes of other datasets with varying degrees of success. They differ from novels, though, in that researchers must often examine data from similar datasets to get the full story about the information they are looking for.

For example, the National Hospital Discharge Survey (NHDS) is a dataset containing hospital discharges for approximately 300,000 patients from about 500 hospitals. These data were obtained from both electronic hospital tapes and transcripts of actual hospital records (Owings and Lawrence, 1999). The Healthcare Cost and Utilization Project-3 (HCUP-3) contains only data obtained from hospital billing systems, but it is composed of a weighted sample of about 8 million hospital stays (Healthcare Cost and Utilization Project, 2006). Both datasets contain information on the total number of discharges by diagnosis. Because the NHDS was in part built using actual hospital transcripts, it contains less nonrandom error than the HCUP-3 dataset. The HCUP-3 is derived from a very large sample; it has less sampling error and contains a larger number of variables that are useful for cost-effectiveness analysis.

When you are looking for one particular variable contained in many datasets, you probably will want to use various values in a sensitivity analysis. Knowing where to find the datasets containing these variables is another issue altogether. Table 12.1 lists the sources of information that researchers typically turn to when in need of commonly used inputs in cost-effectiveness analyses.

Which Source of Data Do You Turn To?

Students often wonder whether it is best to begin a search for a piece of information in the medical literature or start with electronic data. The answer is simple: always obtain as much information as possible about any parameter you are looking for and look to both sources. Before the advent of data extraction tools, student researchers sometimes chose to forgo the task of digging through complicated datasets to find information they were able to easily obtain from the medical literature. Today it is so easy to obtain electronic information that there is no excuse for failing to take a peek at parameters that can quickly be obtained from datasets.

Students also wonder whether data from the medical literature are superior to data from electronic sources or vice versa. When information is available from both

TABLE 12.1. **Datasets Useful for Finding Frequently Needed Cost-Effectiveness Parameters**

Variable	Possible Sources
Prevalence rate	NHIS, medical literature, NHANES
Incidence rate	Medical literature, NHIS (acute diseases only), NHANES, SEER
Mortality rate	Medical literature, Multiple Cause of Death Dataset, Mortality follow back, SEER, WONDER
Risk ratio	Medical literature.
Population data	U.S. Bureau of the Census, WONDER
Disease severity/distribution	NHIS, NHANES, SEER
Medical utilization (number of hospitalizations, outpatient visits, etc.)	HCFA, HCUP-3, Medicaid, MEPS, SEER-Medicare, NAMCS
Cost of medical care	HCFA, medical literature, HCUP-3, Medicaid, NMES, SEER-Medicare, BLS
Cost of transportation, labor, environmental impact	U.S. Bureau of the Census, BLS, medical literature, Internet search engines, University of Michigan

Note: NHIS = National Health Interview Survey; NHANES = National Health and Nutrition Examination Survey; SEER = Surveillance Epidemiology and End Results; HCFA = Health Care Finance Administration; HCUP-3 = Healthcare Cost and Utilization Project-3; MEPS = Medical Expenditure Panel Survey; NAMCS = National Ambulatory Medical Care Survey; BLS = Bureau of Labor Statistics.

published studies and electronic datasets, it is important to weigh the limitations of each source. The medical literature is often the best source of information for data that are difficult to capture in a dataset, such as the incidence rate of a disease or risk ratios. And electronic datasets are often populated with nationally representative information, greatly improving their external validity.

Generally electronic datasets are most useful for obtaining nationally representative costs, medical care utilization rates, and the prevalence of a disease. Published data are often most useful for finding risk ratios and other forms of data that have been analyzed and processed in experimental trials. Datasets have largely been designed to address research needs that are not often met by scientists publishing in the medical literature. For example, while it would be highly unlikely that you would find a nationally representative sample of cholesterol test results for African American women in the medical literature, you would be able to find such information from the National Health and Nutrition Examination Survey (NHANES). Many national agencies have gone one step further in improving the ease of access to these data by developing data extraction tools.

Data Extraction Tools

Most data extraction tools retrieve information about a particular disease using International Classification for Disease (ICD) codes, Clinical Classification Software (CCS) codes, or Diagnosis Related Groups (DRGs). Table 4.2 in Chapter Four describes these codes.

Software that takes you step by step through a problem is often referred to as a wizard. As you proceed through each extraction tool's wizard, you will be asked information about the demographics of the group you are studying, such as age, race, and income; the diagnosis codes you are interested in; and the output that you want. If you did the exercises in the cost chapter, you are familiar with this process. Unfortunately, the categories offered generally cannot be modified, so you are stuck with the age groups and outputs predefined by the tool. Once you have finished, the tool will present you with tables containing the information you need.

The most comprehensive data extraction tool is maintained by the Bureau of the Census. This tool, called the Federal Electronic Research and Review Extraction Tool (FERRET, http://ferret.bls.census.gov), contains both census and health-related datasets. One of the nice features of the FERRET tool is that it allows you to either download any part of a dataset you are interested in or generate cross-tabulations of data. Exhibit 12.3 is a partial listing of available data compilations with extraction tools.

EXHIBIT 12.3. **Some Data Sources for Which Data Extraction Tools Are Available**

National Center for Health Statistics, http://www.cdc.gov/nchs/sets.htm

Centers for Disease Control's Wonder System, http://wonder.cdc.gov/

Healthy People 2010, http://www.cdc.gov/nchs/about/otheract/hpdata2010/aboutdata2010.htm

Data Ferret (Includes free software for PC/Mac), http://www.cdc.gov/nchs/datawh/ferret/ferret.htm

Perhaps the most comprehensive data extraction tool, WONDER, is maintained by the Centers for Disease Control and Prevention (http://wonder.cdc.gov/). This site contains everything from deaths to population data.

TIPS AND TRICKS

The WONDER data system is a good source of information but was poorly organized at the time of publication. Many of the hidden data gems are buried in the DATA2010 system (http://wonder.cdc.gov/data2010/). If you don't find what you are looking for in the main WONDER system, check out the DATA2010 section.

Every data extraction tool has quirks and limitations, but they are generally very easy to use. Students who have never turned on a computer before have produced publication-quality analyses using these tools. Unfortunately, there are few such systems for international data. This is especially tragic in the case of developing countries because fewer researchers have access to statistical software packages. It is perhaps telling that the U.S. government offers many completely redundant software tools for U.S. data (few of which work well) and almost no tools for data sources outside the country.

Using Printed Tabulations of Electronic Data

A simple way to obtain information is with printed tabulations of data. Like most other data extraction tools, data printouts force the researcher to work with the age, race, and gender groupings the publishers see fit to use. If you use a printed data tabulation, the information must be retyped into your spreadsheet program, but when the data needs are minimal, they are much easier to use than unformatted electronic data. The National Center for Health Statistics (NCHS) offers printed information from the National Health Interview Survey (NHIS) and mortality data, as well as other types of data, for free on its Web site (http://www.cdc.gov/nchs). A search engine is available.

Using Datasets Themselves

Students who know how to load datasets into a statistical software package probably won't be reading this section. For the rest of you, it's probably prudent to seek help before attempting to download a dataset and then open it using a statistical software package. However, readers who have extensively used preloaded datasets and are familiar with a particular statistical package will probably be able to use an electronic dataset without help.

Most datasets are now presented in a format called SAS Transport that can be read by major statistical packages, such as SAS, STATA, and SPSS. There is also a commercial application called Stat/Transfer that will not only convert a dataset into a format readable by your software package but will even let the user select the variables. The code book linked to the dataset will help you select the relevant variables.

One caveat to working with datasets is that you must read the documentation in its entirety before working with the data. Many health datasets use complex sampling designs that require familiarity with multiple weighting factors and also require special software. At the time this book was printed, STATA and SUDAAN were the most robust packages for dealing with complex sample designs, but SPSS could handle datasets using complex sample designs with minor limitations.

For readers from low-income nations or without institutional support, a statistical package simply called R works on all major operating systems and is free. In fact, when using LINUX or Mac OS X, it is now possible to obtain all software needed for data analysis for free. Unfortunately, free statistical packages are a bit trickier to use than commercial applications.

Understanding Error in Electronic Data

Electronic health datasets produced by the U.S. government are usually accompanied by a printed discussion of the limitations of electronic data sources that often includes formulas for evaluating the error that they contain. Occasionally researchers need to use smaller datasets that lack a detailed description of the data limitations. In these instances, it will be necessary to contact one of the authors to discuss the various limitations of the data, including potential sources of nonrandom error.

While the primary limitation of studies in the medical literature is random error, electronic data are more frequently limited by nonrandom error. For example, hospitalization data and mortality data are primarily affected by **misclassification bias**. Misclassification bias arises when the physician who fills out the death certificate writes down the wrong cause of death.

Imagine that a patient developed heart disease as a result of diabetes mellitus. Sometimes the doctor filling out the death certificate is unsure whether to list the diabetes or the heart disease as the cause of death. Therefore, the enumeration of the number of deaths attributed to these medical conditions may be incorrect.

USING UNPUBLISHED DATA

For some cost-effectiveness studies, it will be possible to obtain unpublished data directly from the authors of studies published in the medical literature. Often a research project publishes only selected results of studies, leaving out precisely the information you are looking for. Tracking down the authors of a study is usually simple. Authors may be contacted through the medical journal, the institution with which they are affiliated, or, most easily, using a search engine. Contact information for authors, including institutional affiliations, is published in most medical journals. If you don't get a response, try a coauthor. Sometimes unsolicited e-mails get filtered, so don't give up.

USING DATA FROM PIGGYBACKED STUDIES

Piggybacking is the process of adding an economic evaluation to an existing prospective study (Gold, Siegel, Russell, and Weinstein, 1996; Haddix, Teutsch, Shaffer, and Dunet, 1996). When the primary objective of the study is to collect cost and effectiveness data, the study is sometimes called a **primary cost-effectiveness analysis**.

In these study designs, data on the cost and efficacy of the health intervention under study are collected over the course of the analysis.

Because no single study can capture all of the costs or changes in mortality rates that result from a health intervention, it is usually necessary to supplement the data that the researchers are collecting with information from other studies or from electronic datasets. For example, Bridges and others (2000) examined the efficacy of the influenza vaccine in preventing influenza-like illness while simultaneously collecting information on the number of medical visits, hospitalizations, and medications consumed in the vaccine and placebo arms of their study. They then used the MEDSTAT MarketScan Databases (Medstat, 2006) to estimate the cost of each medical visit and each hospitalization that occurred. With this information, they conducted a cost-benefit analysis of influenza vaccination. Unfortunately, they did not capture costs associated with transmission of the flu virus to high-risk populations.

In addition to problems associated with collecting comprehensive data, the piggyback study design usually cannot directly compare the intervention under study with other potentially useful health interventions for preventing or treating a disease. For example, if a pharmaceutical company wishes to compare the product it is evaluating to other products currently on the market, it would have to add more study arms to the randomized controlled trial, which can be very expensive.

USING EXPERT OPINION

Sometimes information on a parameter is not available through published, electronic, or unpublished sources. When this occurs, the value of the parameter of interest can be estimated using the opinion of experts. Although it would be unusual for a group of experts to correctly guess the true value of a cost-effectiveness input (for example, the number of people a single syphilis patient will infect on average), they will likely be able to guess the highest and lowest possible values for that parameter. When cost-effectiveness data are collected using the opinion of experts, the reference case analysis requires that a formal process be used called the Delphi method. (Discussion of the Delphi method is beyond the scope of this book. I recommend http://www.iit.edu/~it/delphi.html for further reading.)

ORGANIZING YOUR DATA

The bane of any researcher's existence is organizing data. Nevertheless, it is nearly impossible to conduct a research project without a good organizational system. Of course, a good filing system will be necessary to keep track of all of the different medical articles. But it is just as important to keep track of the parameters you will use when it comes time to put all of the information you have collected into a decision analysis model.

There are two major goals to organizing data. The first is to create a summary of each dataset and each study from the medical literature that you will be using. This will allow you to quickly review the benefits or the pitfalls of each data element before using it. The second is to have a source of key data elements you will be using to construct your decision analysis model.

No matter how carefully you read a study or a summary of a dataset, you will forget many of its key elements. Having each dataset and study summarized concisely allows you to refer to it quickly. When the Centers for Disease Control and Prevention set out to summarize the medical literature on community preventive services, it hired a small army of public health students and junior researchers. These students summarized the data from each of the thousands of studies they reviewed so that they could quickly put all of the information together in a way that made sense and so that the authors could easily refer to the materials if they had questions (I was one of those lackeys in my youth). You would do well to heed their example, albeit on a much smaller scale.

APPENDIX

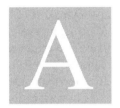

ANSWER KEY TO EXERCISES

CHAPTER 1

1.   The total cost of Staphbegone is $12,000 + $1,000/day × 5 days = $17,000. The total cost of Staphbeilln is $4,000 + $1,000/day × 10 days = $14,000. The incremental cost of Staphbegone is therefore $17,000 − $14,000 = $3,000.

2.   The incremental cost is $17,000 − $14,000 = $3,000, and the incremental effectiveness is 35 QALYs − 34.5 QALYs = 0.5 QALYs. Therefore, the incremental cost-effectiveness is $3,000/0.5 QALYs = $6,000 per QALY gained.

3.   1,000/375/QALY gained = 2.67 QALYs gained.

4.   The mosquito net strategy will purchase $1,000/$846/QALY = 1.18 QALYs. The measles strategy will purchase $1,000/$375/QALY = $2.67 QALYs. The number of QALYs forgone is equal to 2.67 QALYs − 1.18 QALYs = 1.48 QALYs relative to doing nothing.

CHAPTER 2

1.   To calculate the incremental cost-effectiveness ratio for oseltamivir relative to supportive care, the next most effective intervention is subtracted from the most effective intervention. The incremental cost-effectiveness of providing oseltamivir to persons with influenza is ($100 − $10)/(0.5 − 0.1) = ($90/0.4) = $225 per QALY gained.

191

2.   To calculate the incremental cost-effectiveness ratio, the next most effective intervention is subtracted from the most effective intervention. The incremental cost-effectiveness of vaccination relative to treatment is thus ($150 − $100)/(0.75 − 0.5) = $200 per QALY gained.

3.   This question will inform policymakers of the maximum possible benefit that would be realized by vaccinating everyone, with the caveat that it is not likely that the goal will ever be achieved. It will be relevant in instances in which a law is passed requiring people to receive vaccination but will not have much relevance for a recommendation in favor of vaccination that produces only small increases in vaccination rates.

4.   Any costs associated with long-term side effects of the vaccine that affect quality of life. If there is no vaccine-related morbidity that the insurance company might have to pay for, such as side effects from the vaccine, then no morbidity costs are included. However, it may or may not be relevant to include the monetary costs associated with medical care provided to treat minor or short-term side effects. Here, it is critical to distinguish between pain and suffering caused by side effects (morbidity costs) from costs associated with medical care consumed secondary to the side effects (direct costs).

5.   In the numerator. In most cases, the time a patient spends ill with disease (for example, lost productivity and leisure time costs) is captured in the HRQL score. In this case, you will not include an HRQL score in your analysis because you are looking at life years gained rather than QALYs gained. Therefore, you'll want to come up with some value for the time a patient spends while sick. There is no perfect way to measure such a subjective state, but a conservative approach is to include lost wages.

CHAPTER 3

1.   In this question, the critical decision you are asked to make is between what is currently thought to be the best practice and something that may or may not be better. You therefore probably want to know how the new drug compares against the antibiotic that most experts feel is the optimal choice.

CHAPTER 4

1.   First, there is the cost of the patient's time. If the patient spends ten days in the hospital, the value of his or her time can be quite high. Second, there is the cost of transportation to the hospital. This can be high if the patient were brought in an ambulance, for example. Finally, we might think of home care and so on for someone who was sick enough to be hospitalized. There is no 100 percent right answer to this question; it is designed to help you identify some of the costs associated with each event in an event pathway.

2. Using 2003 data, you should have obtained a mean charge of $16,683 for influenza virus infection, ICD-9 code 487. The design of this Web site changes frequently, and hospitals may have been added, so the number you get may differ slightly.

TIPS AND TRICKS

At the time of the printing of this book in 2007, the United States was still using ICD-9 codes for most public datasets. The rest of the world is mostly using ICD-10 codes.

3. This exercise asks you to place a value on the patient's time and add it to the hospital charge you calculated in exercise 2. Again, the numbers you calculate may have changed slightly, but if you got 5.3 days, then the patient time costs are:

$$5.3 \text{ days} \times \$100 \text{ days} = \$530.$$

4. $2,717,280, 218 \div 9,770,496,364 = 0.28.$

5. Cost = Charge $\times$ cost-to-charge ratio = $17,449 \times 0.28 = $4,886.

6. In the table below, we see how costs are inflated from year to year. Note that the correct answer depends on when the original cost of $100 was incurred. If it occurred in January 2002, we would want to inflate the base figure by the 2002 rate of inflation. But here we'll assume it occurred at the end of the year.

Year	Percentage Change	
2002		$100
2003	4.00 percent	$100 \times 0.040 = $104
2004	4.40 percent	$104 \times 0.044 = $109
2005	4.30 percent	$109 \times 0.043 = $113

CHAPTER 5

1. The cost of supportive care = $0.01 \times \$84 = \$0.84$ or about $1. The cost of vaccination is about $0.99 \times \$10 + 0.01 \times \$38 = \$10.28$ or about $10.

2. If that person sees a doctor, she will incur a cost of $12 plus $110 (for the medical visit). This is represented in the Sees Doctor arm as "Cost = Cost + $110." Because the cost up to that point is $12, the variable Cost assumes a total value of $110 + $12 = $122 at this point in the tree. Finally, we must add the cost of hospitalization to this running total. The total value of Cost at the end of this pathway is $12 + $110 + $5,000 = $5,122.

3. Subjects who do not see a doctor and are not subsequently hospitalized incur only the cost of illness, $12.

4.   The average value is the probabilistically weighted mean of the value Cost assumes at each terminal node. ("Probabilistically" weighted means that the cost of each event is multiplied by the probability of incurring that cost, yielding the average cost.) Thus, subjects in the Sees Doctor arm incur a cost of $5,122 × 0.01 + $122 × 0.99 = $172.

CHAPTER 8

1.   You have been told that mortality is reduced by 50 percent. This is equivalent to a risk ratio of 0.5. In the life table, enter 0.5 where it says "Crude RR." You will notice that life expectancy increases from 77.5 to 86.4 years, or a gain of 8.9 years.

2.   The life table provides the average life expectancy for the average American (which is 77.5 years at birth and 22.2 years at age 60). On the spreadsheet, enter 1.1 in each cell for persons over the age of 60. You should see that life expectancy at birth changes to 76.6, and life expectancy at age 60 changes to 21.3. The life expectancy for the average person with diabetes is thus 21.3 years. Those receiving treatment have a 5 percent risk reduction from 1.1, or 1.1 × 0.95 = 1.045. Replacing the 1.1 values with 1.045, you end up with a life expectancy at age 60 of 21.8 years. Thus, your gain in life years at age 60 is 21.8 − 21.3 = 0.5 years of life.

3.   First, calculate QALY for persons at age 60 who are receiving current practice. Enter 1.1 in every risk ratio cell starting at age 60. Next, enter 0.7 in every HRQL score cell beginning at age 60. The QALE at birth should be 71.0 QALYs, and the QALE at age 60 should be 14.9 QALYs. You have a 10 percent improvement in HRQL with treatment, so the mean HRQL among treated persons is 0.7 × 1.1 = 0.77. Don't forget to reenter 1.045 as the risk ratio for treated people. Your new QALE at age 60 is 16.8. Thus, your gain in QALYs is 16.8 − 14.9 = 1.9 QALYs gained at age 60.

4.   The answer varies depending on your country of origins and demographics.

5.   Over the one year of operation, you spend $100,000 on program costs. However, you are also preventing HIV cases. For every HIV case you prevent, you will save $1,000 per year for the rest of each patient's life. Therefore, future HIV costs prevented must be considered over the remaining life of each patient. For instance, preventing a single HIV-positive case who has 5 years of life remaining would reduce future (undiscounted) costs by 15 × $1,000 = $15,000.

6.   HIV-positive people live 15 years. If these 100 cases had become positive, they would have cost $1,000 × 15 years each. This amounts to $15,000 × 100 = $1,500,000 over their lifetimes. Thus, you have saved $1.5 million in future medical costs.

7.   Remember to discount the $1,000 "$t$" years into the future using the formula: $1,000/(1.03)^t$. Thus, year 5 values are $1,000/(1.03)^5$. Savings per patient over 15 years are as follows:

Year	Base Savings	Discounted Savings
1	$1,000	$1,000
2	$1,000	$971
3	$1,000	$943
4	$1,000	$915
5	$1,000	$888
6	$1,000	$863
7	$1,000	$837
8	$1,000	$813
9	$1,000	$789
10	$1,000	$766
11	$1,000	$744
12	$1,000	$722
13	$1,000	$701
14	$1,000	$681
15	$1,000	$661
Sum	$15,000	$12,296

Thus, the total savings are $100 \times \$12,296 = \$1,229,600$.

8.

Year	QALYs	Discounted QALYs
1	0.6	0.6
2	0.6	0.58
3	0.6	0.57
4	0.6	0.55
5	0.6	0.53
6	0.6	0.52
7	0.6	0.50
8	0.6	0.49
9	0.6	0.47
10	0.6	0.46
11	0.6	0.45
12	0.6	0.43
13	0.6	0.42
14	0.6	0.41
15	0.6	0.40
Sum	9.00	7.38

9.

	HIV Positive		HIV Negative	
Year	QALYs	Discounted QALYs	QALYs	Discounted QALYs
1	0.6	0.6	0.9	0.9
2	0.6	0.58	0.9	0.87
3	0.6	0.57	0.9	0.85
4	0.6	0.55	0.9	0.82
5	0.6	0.53	0.9	0.80
6	0.6	0.52	0.9	0.78
7	0.6	0.50	0.9	0.75
8	0.6	0.49	0.9	0.73
9	0.6	0.47	0.9	0.71
10	0.6	0.46	0.9	0.69
11	0.6	0.45	0.9	0.67
12	0.6	0.43	0.9	0.65
13	0.6	0.42	0.9	0.63
14	0.6	0.41	0.9	0.61
15	0.6	0.40	0.9	0.60
Sum	9.00	7.38	13.50	11.07

CHAPTER 9

1. $20.92 and $41.82.

APPENDIX

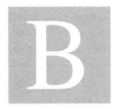

LIFE EXPECTANCY AND QUALITY-ADJUSTED LIFE EXPECTANCY TABLES

TABLE B.1. **Abridged Life Table for the Total Population, 2003**

Age	Probability of Dying Between Ages X and X + N	Number Surviving to Age X	Number Dying Between Ages X and X + N	Person-Years Lived Between Ages X and X + N	Total Number of Person-Years Lived Above Age X	Expectancy of Life at Age X
0–1	0.006865	100,000	687	99,394	7,748,865	77.5
1–5	0.001252	99,313	124	396,962	7,649,471	77.0
5–10	0.000734	99,189	73	495,756	7,252,510	73.1
10–15	0.000956	99,116	95	495,369	6,756,754	68.2
15–20	0.003317	99,022	328	494,435	6,261,385	63.2
20–25	0.004806	98,693	474	492,277	5,766,950	58.4
25–30	0.004751	98,219	467	489,938	5,274,672	53.7
30–35	0.005541	97,752	542	487,457	4,784,734	48.9
35–40	0.007886	97,210	767	484,249	4,297,277	44.2
40–45	0.011992	96,444	1,157	479,513	3,813,027	39.5
45–50	0.017862	95,287	1,702	472,435	3,333,515	35.0
50–55	0.025653	93,585	2,401	462,242	2,861,080	30.6
55–60	0.037558	91,185	3,425	447,912	2,398,838	26.3
60–65	0.058021	87,760	5,092	426,797	1,950,925	22.2
65–70	0.086287	82,668	7,133	396,471	1,524,128	18.4
70–75	0.130072	75,535	9,825	354,252	1,127,657	14.9
75–80	0.197364	65,710	12,969	297,321	773,405	11.8
80–85	0.298685	52,741	15,753	224,973	476,084	9.0
85–90	0.423047	36,988	15,648	145,292	251,112	6.8
90–95	0.579341	21,340	12,363	73,760	105,820	5.0
95–100	0.736793	8,977	6,614	26,017	32,060	3.6
100 +	1.000000	2,363	2,363	6,044	6,044	2.6

Source: Centers for Disease Control and Prevention, National Center for Health Statistics.

TABLE B.2. Life Expectancy at Selected Ages by Race and Sex. United States, 2003

Exact Age in Years	All Races[a]			White			Black		
	Both Sexes	Male	Female	Both Sexes	Male	Female	Both Sexes	Male	Female
0	77.5	74.8	80.1	78.0	75.3	80.5	72.7	69.0	76.1
1	77.0	74.3	79.6	77.4	74.8	79.9	72.7	69.1	76.0
5	73.1	70.4	75.7	73.5	70.9	76.0	68.9	65.3	72.2
10	68.2	65.5	70.7	68.5	66.0	71.0	63.9	60.3	67.2
15	63.2	60.6	65.8	63.6	61.0	66.1	59.0	55.4	62.3
20	58.4	55.8	60.9	58.8	56.3	61.2	54.2	50.7	57.4
25	53.7	51.2	56.0	54.1	51.6	56.3	49.6	46.3	52.6
30	48.9	46.5	51.2	49.3	46.9	51.5	45.0	41.8	47.8
35	44.2	41.9	46.4	44.5	42.2	46.6	40.4	37.3	43.1
40	39.5	37.3	41.6	39.8	37.6	41.9	36.0	32.9	38.6
45	35.0	32.8	37.0	35.2	33.1	37.2	31.6	28.7	34.1
50	30.6	28.5	32.4	30.8	28.8	32.6	27.6	24.8	29.9
55	26.3	24.4	28.0	26.5	24.6	28.1	23.8	21.2	25.9
60	22.2	20.4	23.8	22.3	20.6	23.8	20.2	17.9	22.1
65	18.4	16.8	19.8	18.5	16.9	19.8	17.0	14.9	18.5
70	14.9	13.5	16.0	14.9	13.5	16.0	14.0	12.1	15.3
75	11.8	10.5	12.6	11.7	10.5	12.6	11.4	9.8	12.4
80	9.0	8.0	9.6	9.0	8.0	9.6	9.2	7.9	9.8
85	6.8	6.0	7.2	6.7	5.9	7.1	7.4	6.4	7.8
90	5.0	4.4	5.2	4.9	4.3	5.1	5.7	5.0	6.0
95	3.6	3.2	3.7	3.5	3.1	3.6	4.4	3.8	4.5
100	2.6	2.3	2.6	2.5	2.2	2.5	3.4	3.0	3.4

[a]Includes races other than white and black.

TABLE B.3. Abridged Quality-Adjusted Life Table for the Total Population, 2003

Age	Probability of Dying Between Ages X and X+N	Number Surviving to Age X	Number Dying Between Ages X and X+N	Person-Years Lived Between Ages X and X+N	HRQL Score[a]	Quality-Adjusted Person-Years Lived Between Ages X and X+N	Total Number of Quality-Adjusted Person-Years Lived Above Age X	Quality Adjusted Life Expectancy at Age X
0–1	0.006865	100,000	687	99,394	0.94	93,430	6,359,500	63.6
1–5	0.001252	99,313	124	396,962	0.94	373,144	6,266,070	63.1
5–10	0.000734	99,189	73	495,756	0.93	461,053	5,892,926	59.4
10–15	0.000956	99,116	95	495,369	0.93	460,693	5,431,873	54.8
15–20	0.003317	99,022	328	494,435	0.92	454,880	4,971,180	50.2
20–25	0.004806	98,693	474	492,277	0.89	438,151	4,516,300	45.8
25–30	0.004751	98,219	467	489,938	0.84	409,139	4,078,149	41.5
30–35	0.005541	97,752	542	487,457	0.84	407,067	3,669,010	37.5
35–40	0.007886	97,210	767	484,249	0.84	404,388	3,261,943	33.6
40–45	0.011992	96,444	1,157	479,513	0.84	400,432	2,857,555	29.6
45–50	0.017862	95,287	1,702	472,435	0.84	394,522	2,457,123	25.8
50–55	0.025653	93,585	2,401	462,242	0.79	365,318	2,062,601	22.0
55–60	0.037558	91,185	3,425	447,912	0.73	328,665	1,697,283	18.6
60–65	0.058021	87,760	5,092	426,797	0.73	313,171	1,368,618	15.6
65–70	0.086287	82,668	7,133	396,471	0.73	290,919	1,055,447	12.8
70–75	0.130072	75,535	9,825	354,252	0.73	259,940	764,528	10.1
75–80	0.197364	65,710	12,969	297,321	0.65	193,979	504,589	7.7
80–85	0.298685	52,741	15,753	224,973	0.65	146,778	310,609	5.9
85–90	0.423047	36,988	15,648	145,292	0.65	94,792	163,831	4.4
90–95	0.579341	21,340	12,363	73,760	0.65	48,123	69,039	3.2
95–100	0.736793	8,977	6,614	26,017	0.65	16,974	20,917	2.3
100 +	1.000000	2,363	2,363	6,044	0.65	3,943	3,943	1.7

Source: Centers for Disease Control and Prevention, National Center for Health Statistics and Agency for Health Research and Quality.

[a]HRQL scores obtained from Medical Expenditure Panel Survey. Scores for subjects aged 0 to 18 from Erickson, Wilson, and Shannon (1995).

APPENDIX

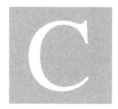

EUROQOL INSTRUMENT AND WEIGHTING SCHEME

Instructions: Responses to the form check boxes correspond to the values listed in the table provided. For subjects residing in the United States, the form is scored by subtracting the corresponding numbers from 1.0. For subjects in the United Kingdom, it's necessary to subtract 0.081 if any value is above 0. If any value is above 3, it is necessary to both subtract 0.081 and add 0.269.

By placing a check in one box in each group, please indicate which statements best describe your own health state today.

EXHIBIT 1. EuroQol 5D Health Domains

Mobility

I have no problems in walking about	☐
I have some problems in walking about	☐
I am confined to bed	☐

Self-Care

I have no problems with self-care	☐
I have some problems washing or dressing myself	☐
I am unable to wash or dress myself	☐

Usual Activities (*e.g., work, study, housework, family, or leisure activities*)

I have no problems with performing my usual activities	☐
I have some problems with performing my usual activities	☐
I am unable to perform my usual activities	☐

Pain/Discomfort

I have no pain or discomfort	☐
I have moderate pain or discomfort	☐
I have extreme pain or discomfort	☐

Anxiety/Depression

I am not anxious or depressed	☐
I am moderately anxious or depressed	☐
I am extremely anxious or depressed	☐

Scoring the EuroQol

	No Problems (Response 1)	Some Problems (Response 2)	Severe Problems/ Inability (Response 3)
United States			
Mobility	0	0.146	0.558
Self-Care	0	0.175	0.471
Usual Activities	0	0.14	0.374
Pain/Discomfort	0	0.173	0.537
Anxiety/Depression	0	0.156	0.45

Formula: 1 − weighting sum

	No Problems (Response 1)	Some Problems (Response 2)	Severe Problems/ Inability (Response 3)
United Kingdom			
Mobility	0	0.069	0.314
Self-Care	0	0.104	0.214
Usual Activities	0	0.036	0.094
Pain/Discomfort	0	0.123	0.386
Anxiety/Depression	0	0.071	0.236

Formula: If no scores are above 3: 1 − (0.081 − weighting sum)
If at least one score is above 3: 1 − (0.081 − weighting sum + 0.269)

APPENDIX

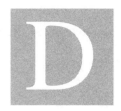

DIAGNOSIS, CHARGES, MEDICARE REIMBURSEMENT, AVERAGE LENGTH OF STAY, AND COST-TO-CHARGE RATIO BY DIAGNOSIS-RELATED GROUPS, 2004

Source: Based on MEDPAR Inpatient Hospital National Data for Fiscal Year 2004.

	1	2	3	4	5
				Average Length of Stay	Cost to
DRG[A]	Diagnosis	Covered Charges	Medicare Reimbursement	(Days)	Charge
001	SURG CRANIOTOMY AGE > 17 W CC	$1,915,759,780	$623,270,066	10.3	0.33
002	SURG CRANIOTOMY AGE > 17 W/O CC	$435,948,632	$133,227,638	4.7	0.31
003	SURG CRANIOTOMY AGE 0–17	—	—	—	—
004	SURG NO LONGER VALID	—	—	—	—
005	SURG NO LONGER VALID	—	—	—	—
006	SURG CARPAL TUNNEL RELEASE	$5,841,970	$1,666,740	3.1	0.29
007	SURG PERIPH & CRANIAL NERVE & OTHER NERV SYST PROC	$747,454,594	$235,845,327	9.4	0.32
008	SURG PERIPH & CRANIAL NERVE & OTHER NERV SYST PROC	$108,028,889	$31,139,646	2.9	0.29
009	MED SPINAL DISORDERS & INJURIES	$55,309,546	$16,928,886	6.9	0.31
010	MED NERVOUS SYSTEM NEOPLASMS W CC	$442,157,226	$135,438,905	6.1	0.31
011	MED NERVOUS SYSTEM NEOPLASMS W/O CC	$52,444,406	$14,333,546	3.8	0.27
012	MED DEGENERATIVE NERVOUS SYSTEM DISORDERS	$1,427,122,662	$507,032,426	7.9	0.36
013	MED MULTIPLE SCLEROSIS & CEREBELLAR ATAXIA	$120,926,162	$32,017,062	5.1	0.26

DRG[A]	Diagnosis	1 Covered Charges	2 Medicare Reimbursement	3 Average Length of Stay (Days)	4 Cost to Charge	5
014	MED INTRACRA- NIAL HEMORRHAGE & STROKE W INFARCT	$5,244,346,417	$1,495,065,981	5.7	0.29	
015	MED NONSPECIFIC CVA & PRECEREBRAL OCCLUSION W/O IN	$382,308,297	$108,316,471	6.4	0.28	
016	MED NONSPECIFIC CEREBROVASCULAR DISORDERS W CC	$1,242,328,339	$355,296,257	4.6	0.29	
017	MED NONSPECIFIC CEREBROVASCULAR DISORDERS W/O CC	$39,280,541	$9,683,111	3.3	0.25	
018	MED CRANIAL & PERIPHERAL NERVE DISORDERS W CC	$586,213,293	$169,134,975	5.3	0.29	
019	MED CRANIAL & PERIPHERAL NERVE DISORDERS W/O CC	$111,254,746	$29,104,460	3.5	0.26	
020	MED NERVOUS SYSTEM INFEC- TION EXCEPT VIRAL MENINGIT	$314,093,777	$101,574,497	9.9	0.32	
021	MED VIRAL MENINGITIS	$57,679,416	$17,703,552	6.3	0.31	
022	MED HYPERTENSIVE ENCEPHALOPATHY	$67,906,393	$17,678,154	5.2	0.26	
023	MED NONTRAUMATIC STUPOR & COMA	$158,184,931	$46,898,790	4.1	0.30	
024	MED SEIZURE & HEAD- ACHE AGE >17 W CC	$1,151,431,252	$331,162,362	4.7	0.29	
025	MED SEIZURE & HEADACHE AGE >17 W/O CC	$326,714,322	$81,906,235	3.1	0.25	
026	MED SEIZURE & HEAD- ACHE AGE 0–17	$814,459	$225,616	5.7	0.28	

(Continued)

	1	2	3	4	5
				Average Length	
			Medicare	of Stay	Cost to
DRG[A]	Diagnosis	Covered Charges	Reimbursement	(Days)	Charge
027	MED TRAUMATIC STUPOR & COMA, COMA >1 HR	$146,280,575	$42,507,400	5.2	0.29
028	MED TRAUMATIC STUPOR & COMA, COMA < 1 HR AGE > 17 W	$435,553,613	$131,085,704	5.9	0.30
029	MED TRAUMATIC STUPOR & COMA, COMA < 1 HR AGE > 17 W/	$86,435,044	$22,135,828	3.4	0.26
030	MED TRAUMATIC STUPOR & COMA, COMA < 1 HR AGE 0–17	—	—	—	—
031	MED CONCUSSION AGE > 17 W CC	$92,629,062	$22,295,901	4	0.24
032	MED CONCUSSION AGE > 17 W/O CC	$23,695,136	$4,536,864	2.4	0.19
033	MED CONCUSSION AGE 0–17	—	—	—	—
034	MED OTHER DISORDERS OF NERVOUS SYSTEM W CC	$522,977,327	$151,486,455	5	0.29
035	MED OTHER DISORDERS OF NERVOUS SYSTEM W/O CC	$95,613,998	$25,907,970	3.2	0.27
036	SURG RETINAL PROCEDURES	$20,806,298	$4,710,736	1.6	0.23
037	SURG ORBITAL PROCEDURES	$30,123,614	$7,934,210	4.2	0.26
038	SURG PRIMARY IRIS PROCEDURES	$731,619	$137,671	3.5	0.19

DRG[A]	Diagnosis	1 Covered Charges	2 Medicare Reimbursement	3 Average Length of Stay (Days)	4 Cost to Charge
039	SURG LENS PROCEDURES WITH OR WITHOUT VITRECTOMY	$6,381,115	$1,537,945	2.4	0.24
040	SURG EXTRAOCULAR PROCEDURES EXCEPT ORBIT AGE > 17	$26,521,235	$7,108,436	4.1	0.27
041	SURG C65 EXTRAOCULAR PROCEDURES EXCEPT ORBIT AGE 0–17	—	—	—	—
042	SURG INTRAOCULAR PROCEDURES EXCEPT RETINA, LENS	$18,241,624	$4,495,172	2.8	0.25
043	MED HYPHEMA	$1,443,607	$341,726	3.1	0.24
044	MED ACUTE MAJOR EYE INFECTIONS	$15,388,777	$3,886,840	4.8	0.25
045	MED NEUROLOGICAL EYE DISORDERS	$38,375,998	$9,712,121	3.1	0.25
046	MED OTHER DISORDERS OF THE EYE AGE > 17 W CC	$53,313,938	$15,284,827	4.2	0.29
047	MED OTHER DISORDERS OF THE EYE AGE > 17 W/O CC	$13,285,058	$3,415,519	3	0.26
048	MED OTHER DISORDERS OF THE EYE AGE 0–17	—	—	—	—
050	SURG MAJOR HEAD & NECK PROCEDURES	$35,441,910	$9,055,690	1.8	0.26
051	SURG SIALOADENECTOMY	$3,200,027	$835,923	2.8	0.26
052	SURG SALIVARY GLAND PROCEDURES EXCEPT SIALOADENECT	$2,615,985	$602,650	2	0.23

(Continued)

	1	2	3	4	5
				Average Length	
			Medicare	of Stay	Cost to
DRG^A	Diagnosis	Covered Charges	Reimbursement	(Days)	Charge
053	SURG CLEFT LIP & PALATE REPAIR	$58,018,998	$15,429,644	4	0.27
054	SURG SINUS & MASTOID PROCE- DURES AGE > 17	—	—	—	—
055	SURG SINUS & MASTOID PROCE- DURES AGE 0–17	$25,681,973	$7,050,253	3.1	0.27
056	SURG MISCELLANE- OUS EAR, NOSE, MOUTH & THROAT PROCE	$7,123,758	$1,983,047	2.6	0.28
057	SURG RHINOPLASTY	$14,695,302	$4,132,736	4.2	0.28
058	SURG T&A PROC, EX- CEPT TONSILLECTOMY &/OR ADENOIDEC	—	—	—	—
059	SURG T&A PROC, EX- CEPT TONSILLECTOMY &/OR ADENOIDEC	$1,516,313	$481,303	2.6	0.32
059	SURG TONSILLECTO- MY &/OR ADENOIDEC- TOMY ONLY, AGE > 17	$84,587,733	$26,519,732	4.4	0.31
060	SURG TONSILLECTOMY &/ OR ADENOIDECTOMY ONLY, AGE 0–17	—	—	—	—
061	SURG MYRINGOTOMY W TUBE INSERTION AGE > 17	$5,307,095	$1,485,102	5.4	0.28
062	SURG MYRINGOTOMY W TUBE INSERTION AGE 0–17	—	—	—	—
063	SURG OTHER EAR, NOSE, MOUTH & THROAT O.R. PROCEDUR	$78,705,234	$23,117,354	4.5	0.29

DRG[A]	Diagnosis	1 Covered Charges	2 Medicare Reimbursement	3 Average Length of Stay (Days)	4 Cost to Charge	5
064	MED EAR, NOSE, MOUTH & THROAT MALIGNANCY	$76,601,471	$26,054,253	6.2	0.34	
065	MED DYSEQUILIBRIUM	$441,255,146	$103,037,985	2.8	0.23	
066	MED EPISTAXIS	$85,629,298	$21,669,833	3.1	0.25	
067	MED EPIGLOTTITIS	$5,728,957	$1,536,963	3.7	0.27	
068	MED OTITIS MEDIA & URI AGE > 17 W CC	$200,661,499	$50,291,287	4	0.25	
069	MED OTITIS MEDIA & URI AGE > 17 W/O CC	$40,551,492	$9,380,559	3	0.23	
070	MED OTITIS MEDIA & URI AGE 0–17	$246,754	$38,606	2.3	0.16	
071	MED LARYNGOTRA-CHEITIS	$886,624	$210,675	4	0.24	
072	MED NASAL TRAUMA & DEFORMITY	$14,893,664	$3,620,460	3.4	0.24	
073	MED OTHER EAR, NOSE, MOUTH & THROAT DIAGNOSES AGE 17	$118,625,813	$32,034,603	4.4	0.27	
074	MED OTHER EAR, NOSE, MOUTH & THROAT DIAGNOSES AGE 0–17	—	—	—	—	
075	SURG MAJOR CHEST PROCEDURES	$2,510,349,050	$798,495,409	9.7	0.32	
076	SURG OTHER RESP SYSTEM O.R. PROCEDURES W CC	$2,384,744,710	$757,227,995	10.8	0.32	
077	SURG OTHER RESP SYSTEM O.R. PROCEDURES W/O CC	$46,514,754	$13,825,323	4.6	0.30	
078	MED PULMONARY EMBOLISM	$972,199,550	$293,535,777	6.3	0.30	

(Continued)

	1	2	3	4	5
DRG[A]	Diagnosis	Covered Charges	Medicare Reimbursement	Average Length of Stay (Days)	Cost to Charge
079	MED RESPIRATORY INFECTIONS & INFLAM- MATIONS AGE > 17	$4,679,657,164	$1,417,207,729	8.2	0.30
080	MED RESPIRATORY INFECTIONS & INFLAM- MATIONS AGE > 17	$118,144,755	$31,028,547	5.4	0.26
081	MED RESPIRATORY IN- FECTIONS & INFLAM- MATIONS AGE 0–17	—	—	—	—
082	MED RESPIRATORY NEOPLASMS	$1,610,496,169	$476,048,784	6.7	0.30
083	MED MAJOR CHEST TRAUMA W CC	$121,211,382	$30,637,616	5.2	0.25
084	MED MAJOR CHEST TRAUMA W/O CC	$15,442,696	$2,941,637	3.1	0.19
085	MED PLEURAL EFFUSION W CC	$473,397,440	$136,662,649	6.2	0.29
086	MED PLEURAL EFFUSION W/O CC	$22,844,389	$6,085,750	3.6	0.27
087	MED PULMONARY EDEMA & RESPIRA- TORY FAILURE	$1,917,733,060	$556,204,871	6.5	0.29
088	MED CHRONIC OBSTRUCTIVE PULMONARY DISEASE	$6,296,378,028	$1,725,088,230	4.9	0.27
089	MED SIMPLE PNEUMONIA & PLEURISY AGE > 17 W CC	$9,770,496,364	$2,717,280,218	5.7	0.28
090	MED SIMPLE PNEUMONIA & PLEU- RISY AGE > 17 W/O CC	$480,869,865	$116,840,753	3.8	0.24

	1	2	3	4	5
				Average Length	
				of Stay	Cost to
			Medicare	(Days)	Charge
DRG[A]	Diagnosis	Covered Charges	Reimbursement		
091	MED SIMPLE PNEUMONIA & PLEURISY AGE 0–17	$931,078	$218,635	4.1	0.23
092	MED INTERSTITIAL LUNG DISEASE W CC	$342,581,312	$101,349,545	6	0.30
093	MED INTERSTITIAL LUNG DISEASE W/O CC	$20,181,329	$5,528,266	3.8	0.27
094	MED PNEUMOTHO-RAX W CC	$266,694,225	$74,639,254	6.1	0.28
095	MED PNEUMOTHO-RAX W/O CC	$17,469,473	$4,294,266	3.6	0.25
096	MED BRONCHITIS & ASTHMA AGE > 17 W CC	$752,064,031	$196,039,445	4.4	0.26
097	MED BRONCHITIS & ASTHMA AGE > 17 W/O CC	$254,243,573	$61,235,889	3.4	0.24
098	MED BRONCHITIS & ASTHMA AGE 0–17	—	—	—	—
099	MED RESPIRATORY SIGNS & SYMPTOMS W CC	$271,230,910	$72,282,364	3.1	0.27
100	MED RESPIRATORY SIGNS & SYMPTOMS W/O CC	$65,568,570	$15,218,732	2.1	0.23
101	MED OTHER RES-PIRATORY SYSTEM DIAGNOSES W CC	$359,352,942	$99,043,109	4.3	0.28
102	MED OTHER RESPIRA-TORY SYSTEM DIAG-NOSES W/O CC	$51,611,866	$12,248,502	2.5	0.24
103	RE SURG HEART TRANSPLANT	$215,928,548	$75,475,941	37.1	0.35

(Continued)

	1	2	3	4	5
DRG[A]	Diagnosis	Covered Charges	Medicare Reimbursement	Average Length of Stay (Days)	Cost to Charge
104	SURG CARDIAC VALVE & OTH MAJOR CARDI-OTHORACIC PROC	$3,028,852,231	$1,006,923,853	14.5	0.33
105	SURG CARDIAC VALVE & OTH MAJOR CARDI-OTHORACIC PROC	$3,376,390,980	$1,081,698,129	9.9	0.32
106	SURG CORONARY BYPASS W PTCA	$437,301,551	$141,220,763	11.2	0.32
107	SURG CORONARY BYPASS W CARDIAC CATH	$6,582,013,332	$2,041,744,808	10.5	0.31
108	SURG OTHER CARDIOTHORACIC PROCEDURES	$858,684,059	$280,197,296	9.8	0.33
109	SURG CORONARY BYPASS W/O PTCA OR CARDIAC CATH	$3,589,212,303	$1,097,521,432	7.8	0.31
110	SURG MAJOR CARDIOVASCULAR PROCEDURES W CC	$4,031,674,178	$1,326,203,457	8.4	0.33
111	SURG MAJOR CARDIOVASCULAR PROCEDURES W/O CC	$449,560,706	$132,158,993	3.4	0.29
112	SURG NO LONGER VALID	—	—	—	—
113	SURG AMPUTATION FOR CIRC SYSTEM DISORDERS EXCEPT U	$1,914,138,831	$561,997,190	12.6	0.29
114	SURG UPPER LIMB & TOE AMPUTATION FOR CIRC SYSTEM D	$252,852,619	$77,244,115	8.5	0.31
115	SURG PRM CARD PACEM IMPL W AMI/HR/SHOCK OR AICD LE	$1,424,683,856	$434,936,333	6.8	0.31

	1	2	3	4	5
DRG^A	Diagnosis	Covered Charges	Medicare Reimbursement	Average Length of Stay (Days)	Cost to Charge
116	SURG OTHER PERMANENT CARDIAC PACEMAKER IMPLANT	$4,797,373,475	$1,469,887,869	4.3	0.31
117	SURG CARDIAC PACEMAKER REVISION EXCEPT DEVICE REPL	$123,306,214	$38,642,059	4.2	0.31
118	SURG CARDIAC PACEMAKER DEVICE REPLACEMENT	$227,760,060	$65,638,210	3	0.29
119	SURG VEIN LIGATION & STRIPPING	$24,462,530	$7,495,047	5.5	0.31
120	SURG OTHER CIRCULATORY SYSTEM O.R. PROCEDURES	$1,567,601,857	$490,749,040	9	0.31
121	MED CIRCULATORY DISORDERS W AMI & MAJOR COMP, DISC	$4,284,939,086	$1,246,763,783	6.3	0.29
122	MED CIRCULATORY DISORDERS W AMI W/O MAJOR COMP, DI	$1,014,852,583	$285,727,901	3.4	0.28
123	MED CIRCULATORY DISORDERS W AMI, EXPIRED	$936,439,516	$282,694,676	4.8	0.30
124	MED CIRCULATORY DISORDERS EXCEPT AMI, W CARD CATH	$3,340,825,272	$948,070,922	4.4	0.28
125	MED CIRCULATORY DISORDERS EXCEPT AMI, W CARD CATH	$1,848,826,816	$500,484,357	2.7	0.27
126	MED ACUTE & SUBACUTE ENDOCARDITIS	$272,502,376	$83,285,779	11.3	0.31
127	MED HEART FAILURE & SHOCK	$12,568,243,307	$3,525,378,157	5.1	0.28

(Continued)

DRG[A]	Diagnosis	1 Covered Charges	2 Medicare Reimbursement	3 Average Length of Stay (Days)	4	5 Cost to Charge
128	MED DEEP VEIN THROMBOPHLEBITIS	$62,937,147	$17,303,229	5.2		0.27
129	MED CARDIAC ARREST, UNEXPLAINED	$69,982,852	$19,564,692	2.6		0.28
130	MED PERIPH-ERAL VASCULAR DISORDERS W CC	$1,489,009,708	$425,906,597	5.5		0.29
131	MED PERIPHERAL VASCULAR DISOR-DERS W/O CC	$233,777,868	$59,154,205	3.8		0.25
132	MED ATHEROSCLERO-SIS W CC	$1,279,889,449	$339,545,036	2.8		0.27
133	MED ATHEROSCLERO-SIS W/O CC	$71,208,737	$18,703,844	2.2		0.26
134	MED HYPERTENSION	$462,204,167	$112,592,354	3.1		0.24
135	MED CARDIAC CON-GENITAL & VALVULAR DISORDERS AGE > 17	$123,910,755	$38,522,805	4.5		0.31
136	MED CARDIAC CON-GENITAL & VALVULAR DISORDERS AGE > 17	$13,288,006	$3,160,947	2.8		0.24
137	MED CARDIAC CON-GENITAL & VALVULAR DISORDERS AGE 0–17	—	—	—		—
138	MED CARDIAC AR-RHYTHMIA & CON-DUCTION DISORDERS W CC	$3,021,550,963	$828,390,642	3.9		0.27
139	MED CARDIAC ARRHYTHMIA & CONDUCTION DISORDERS W/O	$724,530,368	$167,249,721	2.4		0.23
140	MED ANGINA PECTORIS	$337,319,439	$83,078,363	2.4		0.25

	1	2	3	4	5
				Average Length	
			Medicare	of Stay	Cost to
DRGᴬ	Diagnosis	Covered Charges	Reimbursement	(Days)	Charge
141	MED SYNCOPE & COLLAPSE W CC	$1,646,527,103	$436,787,228	3.5	0.27
142	MED SYNCOPE & COLLAPSE W/O CC	$555,511,782	$134,340,696	2.5	0.24
143	MED CHEST PAIN	$2,503,782,726	$590,394,957	2.1	0.24
144	MED OTHER CIRCULATORY SYSTEM DIAGNOSES W CC	$2,292,060,028	$667,786,138	5.7	0.29
145	MED OTHER CIR-CULATORY SYSTEM DIAGNOSES W/O CC	$66,104,437	$16,755,411	2.6	0.25
146	SURG RECTAL RESECTION W CC	$500,965,336	$160,372,442	9.9	0.32
147	SURG RECTAL RESECTION W/O CC	$69,459,603	$20,775,337	5.8	0.30
148	SURG MAJOR SMALL & LARGE BOWEL PROCEDURES W CC	$8,061,787,214	$2,615,862,812	12.1	0.32
149	SURG MAJOR SMALL & LARGE BOWEL PROCEDURES W/O CC	$501,320,264	$144,229,840	5.9	0.29
150	SURG PERITONEAL ADHESIOLYSIS W CC	$1,104,667,769	$353,348,400	10.9	0.32
151	SURG PERITONEAL ADHESIOLYSIS W/O CC	$119,726,369	$34,032,299	5.1	0.28
152	SURG MINOR SMALL & LARGE BOWEL PRO-CEDURES W CC	$167,949,965	$52,024,189	8	0.31
153	SURG MINOR SMALL & LARGE BOWEL PRO-CEDURES W/O CC	$40,978,992	$12,040,137	5	0.29

(Continued)

	1	2	3	4	5
				Average Length	
			Medicare	of Stay	Cost to
DRG[A]	Diagnosis	Covered Charges	Reimbursement	(Days)	Charge
154	SURG STOMACH, ESOPHAGEAL & DUO-DENAL PROCEDURES AGE > 17	$2,065,833,700	$688,935,668	13.1	0.33
155	SURG STOMACH, ESOPHAGEAL & DUO-DENAL PROCEDURES AGE > 17	$146,787,064	$40,895,051	4.2	0.28
156	SURG STOMACH, ESOPHAGEAL & DUO-DENAL PROCEDURES AGE 0–17	—	—	—	—
157	SURG ANAL & STOMAL PROCEDURES W CC	$195,248,858	$56,262,939	5.7	0.29
158	SURG ANAL & STOMAL PROCEDURES W/O CC	$49,134,370	$11,488,571	2.6	0.23
159	SURG HERNIA PROCEDURES EXCEPT INGUINAL & FEMORAL A	$481,636,634	$134,045,938	5.1	0.28
160	SURG HERNIA PROCEDURES EXCEPT INGUINAL & FEMORAL A	$178,786,803	$43,876,962	2.7	0.25
161	SURG INGUINAL & FEMORAL HERNIA PRO-CEDURES AGE > 17	$220,611,770	$60,630,371	4.4	0.27
162	SURG INGUINAL & FEMORAL HERNIA PRO-CEDURES AGE > 17	$65,853,641	$15,095,530	2.1	0.23

	1	2	3	4	5
DRG[A]	**Diagnosis**	**Covered Charges**	**Medicare Reimbursement**	**Average Length of Stay (Days)**	**Cost to Charge**
163	SURG HERNIA PROCE-DURES AGE 0–17	$168,223	$45,790	3	0.27
164	SURG APPENDECTO-MY W COMPLICATED PRINCIPAL DIAG W C	$234,227,682	$71,227,927	8	0.30
165	SURG APPENDECTO-MY W COMPLICATED PRINCIPAL DIAG W/O	$52,606,372	$14,466,646	4.2	0.27
166	SURG APPEN-DECTOMY W/O COMPLICATED PRINCIPAL DIAG W	$124,674,684	$34,320,387	4.5	0.28
167	SURG APPEN-DECTOMY W/O COMPLICATED PRINCIPAL DIAG W	$72,640,335	$18,151,828	2.2	0.25
168	SURG MOUTH PROCEDURES W CC	$38,279,144	$11,816,631	4.9	0.31
169	SURG MOUTH PROCEDURES W/O CC	$11,615,315	$3,123,569	2.4	0.27
170	SURG OTHER DIGES-TIVE SYSTEM O.R. PROCEDURES W CC	$919,930,773	$289,942,079	10.8	0.32
171	SURG OTHER DIGES-TIVE SYSTEM O.R. PROCEDURES W/O CC	$33,132,134	$9,206,385	4.1	0.28
172	MED DIGESTIVE MALIGNANCY W CC	$853,448,042	$254,555,402	6.9	0.30
173	MED DIGESTIVE MALIGNANCY W/O CC	$34,438,853	$9,660,653	3.6	0.28
174	MED G.I. HEMOR-RHAGE W CC	$4,765,109,503	$1,330,888,562	4.7	0.28
175	MED G.I. HEMOR-RHAGE W/O CC	$328,436,290	$77,327,304	2.9	0.24

(Continued)

DRG[A]	Diagnosis	1 Covered Charges	2 Medicare Reimbursement	3 Average Length of Stay (Days)	4	5 Cost to Charge
176	MED COMPLICATED PEPTIC ULCER	$288,775,543	$81,490,532	5.2		0.28
177	MED UNCOMPLI-CATED PEPTIC ULCER W CC	$138,366,104	$37,883,415	4.4		0.27
178	MED UNCOMPLI-CATED PEPTIC ULCER W/O CC	$36,023,090	$8,881,551	3.1		0.25
179	MED INFLAMMATORY BOWEL DISEASE	$279,831,666	$78,970,614	5.9		0.28
180	MED G.I. OBSTRUC-TION W CC	$1,568,585,926	$438,619,686	5.3		0.28
181	MED G.I. OBSTRUC-TION W/O CC	$255,302,172	$58,216,877	3.3		0.23
182	MED ESOPHAGITIS, GASTROENT & MISC DIGEST DISORDERS	$4,306,527,322	$1,146,667,997	4.4		0.27
183	MED ESOPHAGITIS, GASTROENT & MISC DIGEST DISORDERS	$881,885,232	$208,642,280	2.9		0.24
184	MED ESOPHAGITIS, GASTROENT & MISC DIGEST DISORDERS	$1,228,566	$225,644	3.6		0.18
185	MED DENTAL & ORAL DIS EXCEPT EXTRAC-TIONS & RESTORA	$91,472,348	$25,589,995	4.5		0.28
186	MED DENTAL & ORAL DIS EXCEPT EXTRAC-TIONS & RESTOR	—	—	—		—
187	MED DENTAL EXTRACTIONS & RESTORATIONS	$9,768,626	$2,391,709	4.2		0.24

	1	2	3	4 Average Length of Stay	5
DRG[A]	Diagnosis	Covered Charges	Medicare Reimbursement	(Days)	Cost to Charge
188	MED OTHER DIGESTIVE SYSTEM DIAGNOSES AGE > 17 W CC	$1,833,629,748	$537,263,303	5.6	0.29
189	MED OTHER DIGESTIVE SYSTEM DIAGNOSES AGE > 17 W/O C	$143,826,442	$36,510,662	3.1	0.25
190	MED OTHER DIGESTIVE SYSTEM DIAGNOSES AGE 0–17	$975,822	$364,154	4.3	0.37
191	SURG PANCREAS, LIVER & SHUNT PROCEDURES W CC	$805,282,353	$296,648,803	12.7	0.37
192	SURG PANCREAS, LIVER & SHUNT PROCEDURES W/O CC	$48,023,329	$15,183,910	5.7	0.32
193	SURG BILIARY TRACT PROC EXCEPT ONLY CHOLECYST W OR	$267,201,131	$90,312,020	12	0.34
194	SURG BILIARY TRACT PROC EXCEPT ONLY CHOLECYST W OR	$15,702,927	$4,823,085	6.7	0.31
195	SURG CHOLECYSTEC-TOMY W C.D.E. W CC	$171,214,951	$52,869,695	10.6	0.31
196	SURG CHOLECYSTEC-TOMY W C.D.E. W/O CC	$19,201,673	$5,474,127	5.7	0.29
197	SURG CHOLECYS-TECTOMY EXCEPT BY LAPAROSCOPE W/O C.D	$764,127,944	$237,083,835	9.1	0.31

(Continued)

	1	2	3	4	5
				Average Length	
			Medicare	of Stay	Cost to
DRG[A]	Diagnosis	Covered Charges	Reimbursement	(Days)	Charge
198	SURG CHOLECYS-TECTOMY EXCEPT BY LAPAROSCOPE W/O C.D	$93,784,025	$25,630,492	4.3	0.27
199	SURG HEPATOBILIARY DIAGNOSTIC PROCE-DURE FOR MALIGN	$65,121,012	$20,757,915	9.4	0.32
200	SURG HEPATOBILIARY DIAGNOSTIC PROCE-DURE FOR NON-MA	$45,719,722	$17,153,330	9.6	0.38
201	SURG OTHER HEPATO-BILIARY OR PANCREAS O.R. PROCEDUR	$187,269,993	$60,618,884	13.7	0.32
202	MED CIRRHOSIS & ALCOHOLIC HEPATITIS	$673,884,708	$197,115,828	6.2	0.29
203	MED MALIGNANCY OF HEPATOBIL-IARY SYSTEM OR PANCREAS	$797,350,694	$237,265,797	6.5	0.30
204	MED DISORDERS OF PANCREAS EXCEPT MALIGNANCY	$1,448,956,797	$428,960,322	5.5	0.30
205	MED DISORDERS OF LIVER EXCEPT MALIG, CIRR, ALC HEPA	$702,853,503	$211,846,384	5.9	0.30
206	MED DISORDERS OF LIVER EXCEPT MALIG, CIRR, ALC HEPA	$28,159,140	$7,280,628	3.9	0.26
207	MED DISORDERS OF THE BILIARY TRACT W CC	$746,526,142	$212,153,692	5.2	0.28
208	MED DISORDERS OF THE BILIARY TRACT W/O CC	$119,603,489	$29,668,775	2.9	0.25

	1	2	3	4 Average Length of Stay	5 Cost to
DRG^A	Diagnosis	Covered Charges	Medicare Reimbursement	(Days)	Charge
209	SURG MAJOR JOINT & LIMB REATTACHMENT PROCEDURES OF	$15,785,128,471	$4,598,778,284	4.6	0.29
210	SURG HIP & FEMUR PROCEDURES EXCEPT MAJOR JOINT AGE 17	$4,070,021,371	$1,187,657,703	6.7	0.29
211	SURG HIP & FEMUR PROCEDURES EXCEPT MAJOR JOINT AGE 17	$584,603,047	$161,570,060	4.7	0.28
212	SURG HIP & FEMUR PROCEDURES EXCEPT MAJOR JOINT AGE 0–17	—	—	—	—
213	SURG AMPUTATION FOR MUSCULOSKEL-ETAL SYSTEM & CONN	$355,826,980	$110,563,148	9.1	0.31
214	SURG NO LONGER VALID	—	—	—	—
215	SURG NO LONGER VALID	—	—	—	—
216	SURG BIOPSIES OF MUSCULOSKELETAL SYSTEM & CONNECTI	$614,780,022	$199,260,135	5.9	0.32
217	SURG WND DEBRID & SKN GRFT EXCEPT HAND, FOR MUSCSKE	$963,875,878	$322,804,179	12.6	0.33
218	SURG LOWER EXTREM & HUMER PROC EXCEPT HIP, FOOT, FEM	$839,047,364	$232,715,866	5.5	0.28
219	SURG LOWER EXTREM & HUMER PROC EXCEPT HIP, FOOT, FEM	$396,126,557	$102,283,952	3.1	0.26

(Continued)

	1	2	3	4	5
				Average Length	
			Medicare	of Stay	Cost to
DRG[A]	Diagnosis	Covered Charges	Reimbursement	(Days)	Charge
220	SURG LOWER EXTREM & HUMER PROC EXCEPT HIP, FOOT, FEM	—	—	—	—
221	SURG NO LONGER VALID	—	—	—	—
222	SURG NO LONGER VALID	—	—	—	—
223	SURG MAJOR SHOUL-DER/ELBOW PROC, OR OTHER UPPER EXT	$264,245,426	$66,311,433	3.2	0.25
224	SURG SHOULDER, ELBOW OR FOREARM PROC, EXC MAJOR JOIN	$155,274,115	$36,835,202	1.9	0.24
225	SURG FOOT PROCEDURES	$141,749,759	$38,060,421	5.2	0.27
226	SURG SOFT TISSUE PROCEDURES W CC	$190,535,146	$57,047,011	6.3	0.30
227	SURG SOFT TISSUE PROCEDURES W/O CC	$79,331,488	$20,074,666	2.6	0.25
228	SURG MAJOR THUMB OR JOINT PROC, OR OTH HAND OR WRIS	$55,245,887	$15,361,781	4.1	0.28
229	SURG HAND OR WRIST PROC, EXCEPT MAJOR JOINT PROC,	$15,516,265	$3,832,059	2.5	0.25
230	SURG LOCAL EXCI-SION & REMOVAL OF INT FIX DEVICES O	$61,591,254	$17,939,568	5.6	0.29
231	SURG NO LONGER VALID	—	—	—	—

DRG^A	Diagnosis	1 Covered Charges	2 Medicare Reimbursement	3 Average Length of Stay (Days)	4 Cost to Charge	5
232	SURG ARTHROSCOPY	$12,532,697	$3,299,283	2.8	0.26	
233	SURG OTHER MUS- CULOSKELET SYS & CONN TISS O.R. PROC	$512,056,169	$164,154,501	6.7	0.32	
234	SURG OTHER MUS- CULOSKELET SYS & CONN TISS O.R. PROC	$167,123,074	$45,375,039	2.8	0.27	
235	MED FRACTURES OF FEMUR	$68,914,744	$19,600,323	4.9	0.28	
236	MED FRACTURES OF HIP & PELVIS	$581,431,258	$162,342,376	4.9	0.28	
237	MED SPRAINS, STRAINS, & DISLOCA- TIONS OF HIP, PELVI	$22,349,382	$5,542,532	3.7	0.25	
238	MED OSTEOMYELITIS	$248,810,211	$73,294,088	8.4	0.29	
239	MED PATHOLOGICAL FRACTURES & MUS- CULOSKELETAL & CON	$808,099,732	$227,507,295	6.1	0.28	
240	MED CONNECTIVE TIS- SUE DISORDERS W CC	$328,074,802	$96,321,852	6.7	0.29	
241	MED CONNECTIVE TISSUE DISORDERS W/O CC	$34,187,447	$8,580,070	3.8	0.25	
242	MED SEPTIC ARTHRITIS	$57,562,488	$17,119,635	6.7	0.30	
243	MED MEDICAL BACK PROBLEMS	$1,395,333,776	$366,366,235	4.6	0.26	
244	MED BONE DIS- EASES & SPECIFIC ARTHROPATHIES W CC	$247,995,995	$81,065,872	5.1	0.33	
245	MED BONE DIS- EASES & SPECIFIC ARTHROPATHIES W/O CC	$62,302,699	$21,164,201	3.9	0.34	

(Continued)

	1	2	3	4	5
				Average Length of Stay	Cost to
			Medicare	of Stay	Cost to
DRG^A	Diagnosis	Covered Charges	Reimbursement	(Days)	Charge
246	MED NON-SPECIFIC ARTHROPATHIES	$21,162,488	$7,515,797	4.7	0.36
247	MED SIGNS & SYMPTOMS OF MUSCULOSKELETAL SYSTEM & C	$228,327,931	$58,312,245	3.4	0.26
248	MED TENDONITIS, MYOSITIS & BURSITIS	$238,021,878	$65,677,696	4.9	0.28
249	MED AFTERCARE, MUSCULOSKELETAL SYSTEM & CONNEC-TIVE	$205,778,670	$60,829,959	4.4	0.30
250	MED FX, SPRN, STRN & DISL OF FOREARM, HAND, FOOT A	$52,611,317	$14,301,394	4	0.27
251	MED FX, SPRN, STRN & DISL OF FOREARM, HAND, FOOT A	$18,595,366	$3,978,486	2.8	0.21
252	MED FX, SPRN, STRN & DISL OF FOREARM, HAND, FOOT	—	—	—	—
253	MED FX, SPRN, STRN & DISL OF UPARM, LOWLEG EX FOOT	$344,063,994	$91,877,750	4.6	0.27
254	MED FX, SPRN, STRN & DISL OF UPARM, LOWLEG EX FOOT	$87,251,616	$19,449,097	3.1	0.22
255	MED FX, SPRN, STRN & DISL OF UPARM, LOWLEG EX FOOT	—	—	—	—
256	MED OTHER MUSCU-LOSKELETAL SYSTEM & CONNECTIVE TISS	$110,175,237	$31,027,095	5.1	0.28

	1	2	3	4	5
DRG[A]	**Diagnosis**	**Covered Charges**	**Medicare Reimbursement**	**Average Length of Stay (Days)**	**Cost to Charge**
257	SURG TOTAL MAS-TECTOMY FOR MALIGNANCY W CC	$215,555,007	$56,381,088	2.6	0.26
258	SURG TOTAL MAS-TECTOMY FOR MALIGNANCY W/O CC	$152,653,478	$36,508,761	1.8	0.24
259	SURG SUBTOTAL MASTECTOMY FOR MALIGNANCY W CC	$50,951,026	$13,458,880	2.7	0.26
260	SURG SUBTOTAL MASTECTOMY FOR MALIGNANCY W/O CC	$37,212,731	$8,856,390	1.4	0.24
261	SURG BREAST PROC FOR NON-MALIGNANCY EXCEPT BIOPSY	$28,713,728	$6,887,725	2.2	0.24
262	SURG BREAST BIOPSY & LOCAL EXCISION FOR NON-MALIGN	$11,256,040	$2,980,249	4.8	0.26
263	SURG SKIN GRAFT &/OR DEBRID FOR SKN ULCER OR CELLU	$843,720,812	$270,121,003	10.8	0.32
264	SURG SKIN GRAFT &/OR DEBRID FOR SKN ULCER OR CELLU	$72,066,179	$20,666,965	6.3	0.29
265	SURG SKIN GRAFT &/OR DEBRID EXCEPT FOR SKIN ULCER	$134,684,888	$40,859,483	6.5	0.30
266	SURG SKIN GRAFT &/OR DEBRID EXCEPT FOR SKIN ULCER	$39,941,084	$10,930,246	3.2	0.27

(Continued)

	1	2	3	4	5
				Average Length of Stay (Days)	Cost to Charge
DRG^A	Diagnosis	Covered Charges	Medicare Reimbursement		
267	SURG PERIANAL & PILONIDAL PROCE-DURES	$4,584,838	$1,381,988	4.2	0.30
268	SURG SKIN, SUBCU-TANEOUS TISSUE & BREAST PLASTIC PR	$22,052,831	$6,231,660	3.5	0.28
269	SURG OTHER SKIN, SUBCUT TISS & BREAST PROC W CC	$345,236,318	$103,876,296	8.3	0.30
270	SURG OTHER SKIN, SUBCUT TISS & BREAST PROC W/O CC	$40,790,932	$10,548,628	3.8	0.26
271	MED SKIN ULCERS	$367,360,927	$111,404,288	6.8	0.30
272	MED MAJOR SKIN DISORDERS W CC	$108,195,996	$32,840,064	5.9	0.30
273	MED MAJOR SKIN DISORDERS W/O CC	$13,947,784	$3,985,253	3.7	0.29
274	MED MALIGNANT BREAST DISORDERS W CC	$48,216,754	$14,583,528	6.3	0.30
275	MED MALIGNANT BREAST DISORDERS W/O CC	$2,358,846	$679,295	3.3	0.29
276	MED NON-MALIGANT BREAST DISORDERS	$18,293,914	$4,601,636	4.5	0.25
277	MED CELLULITIS AGE > 17 W CC	$1,723,968,913	$473,390,043	5.5	0.27
278	MED CELLULITIS AGE > 17 W/O CC	$325,255,558	$76,826,925	4.1	0.24
279	MED CELLULITIS AGE–	$210,225	$43,758	5.2	0.21
280	MED TRAUMA TO THE SKIN, SUBCUT TISS & BREAST AGE > 17	$249,331,610	$64,093,832	4	0.26

	1	2	3	4	5
				Average Length	
			Medicare	of Stay	Cost to
DRG^A	Diagnosis	Covered Charges	Reimbursement	(Days)	Charge
281	MED TRAUMA TO THE SKIN, SUBCUT TISS & BREAST AGE > 17	$63,501,349	$14,137,090	2.8	0.22
282	MED TRAUMA TO THE SKIN, SUBCUT TISS & BREAST AGE 0–17	—	—	—	—
283	MED MINOR SKIN DISORDERS W CC	$86,599,328	$23,939,859	4.6	0.28
284	MED MINOR SKIN DISORDERS W/O CC	$15,478,330	$3,356,049	3	0.22
285	SURG AMPUTAT OF LOWER LIMB FOR ENDOCRINE, NUTRIT, &	$285,738,512	$87,843,254	10	0.31
286	SURG ADRENAL & PI-TUITARY PROCEDURES	$102,993,194	$32,796,753	5.5	0.32
287	SURG SKIN GRAFTS & WOUND DEBRID FOR ENDOC, NUTRIT	$204,996,779	$63,993,108	9.9	0.31
288	SURG O.R. PROCE-DURES FOR OBESITY	$393,423,775	$119,765,746	4.1	0.30
289	SURG PARATHYROID PROCEDURES	$120,290,631	$33,081,352	2.5	0.28
290	SURG THYROID PROCEDURES	$180,870,093	$47,721,408	2.1	0.26
291	SURG THYROGLOSSAL PROCEDURES	$1,389,015	$220,957	2.8	0.16
292	SURG OTHER ENDOCRINE, NUTRIT & METAB O.R. PROC W	$347,639,562	$116,021,539	10	0.33
293	SURG OTHER EN-DOCRINE, NUTRIT & METAB O.R. PROC W/	$9,399,799	$2,745,130	4.6	0.29
294	MED DIABETES AGE > 35	$1,366,367,234	$380,170,175	4.3	0.28

(Continued)

	1	2	3	4	5
			Medicare	Average Length of Stay	Cost to
DRG[A]	**Diagnosis**	**Covered Charges**	**Reimbursement**	**(Days)**	**Charge**
295	MED DIABETES AGE 0–35	$57,541,790	$17,269,621	3.7	0.30
296	MED NUTRITIONAL & MISC METABOLIC DIS-ORDERS AGE > 17	$3,675,886,081	$1,076,865,014	4.7	0.29
297	MED NUTRITIONAL & MISC METABOLIC DIS-ORDERS AGE > 17	$392,589,467	$97,700,210	3.1	0.25
298	MED NUTRITIONAL & MISC METABOLIC DIS-ORDERS AGE 0–17	$1,048,873	$260,543	3.8	0.25
299	MED INBORN ERRORS OF METABOLISM	$26,518,600	$7,280,204	5.2	0.27
300	MED ENDOCRINE DISORDERS W CC	$416,991,885	$124,083,172	5.9	0.30
301	MED ENDOCRINE DISORDERS W/O CC	$43,902,243	$11,690,589	3.4	0.27
302	SURG KIDNEY TRANSPLANT	$1,137,666,421	$215,781,513	8.2	0.19
303	SURG KIDNEY, URETER & MAJOR BLADDER PROCEDURES FOR	$1,004,328,884	$328,143,617	7.4	0.33
304	SURG KIDNEY, URETER & MAJOR BLADDER PROC FOR NON-N	$610,648,402	$197,795,180	8.5	0.32
305	SURG KIDNEY, URETER & MAJOR BLADDER PROC FOR NON-N	$67,645,082	$19,522,741	3.2	0.29
306	SURG PROSTATEC-TOMY W CC	$144,093,665	$39,390,245	5.5	0.27
307	SURG PROSTATEC-TOMY W/O CC	$22,469,684	$5,388,271	2.1	0.24

	1	2	3	4	5
				Average Length	
			Medicare	of Stay	Cost to
DRG^A	Diagnosis	Covered Charges	Reimbursement	(Days)	Charge
308	SURG MINOR BLADDER PROCEDURES W CC	$205,441,020	$60,803,904	6.1	0.30
309	SURG MINOR BLADDER PROCEDURES W/O CC	$58,368,268	$14,874,161	2	0.25
310	SURG TRANSURETHRAL PROCEDURES W CC	$553,218,307	$151,711,819	4.5	0.27
311	SURG TRANSURETHRAL PROCEDURES W/O CC	$74,608,345	$17,891,555	1.9	0.24
312	SURG URETHRAL PROCEDURES, AGE > 17 W CC	$30,864,844	$8,488,225	4.8	0.28
313	SURG URETHRAL PROCEDURES, AGE > 17 W/O CC	$6,702,328	$1,741,166	2.2	0.26
314	SURG URETHRAL PROCEDURES, AGE 0–17	—	—	—	—
315	SURG OTHER KIDNEY & URINARY TRACT O.R. PROCEDURES	$1,401,516,502	$432,149,886	6.8	0.31
316	MED RENAL FAILURE	$4,066,807,831	$1,266,465,020	6.3	0.31
317	MED ADMIT FOR RENAL DIALYSIS	$39,385,712	$12,108,940	3.5	0.31
318	MED KIDNEY & URINARY TRACT NEOPLASMS W CC	$129,057,061	$39,193,999	5.8	0.30
319	MED KIDNEY & URINARY TRACT NEOPLASMS W/O CC	$5,089,095	$1,512,936	2.8	0.30
320	MED KIDNEY & URINARY TRACT INFECTIONS AGE > 17 W C	$3,319,507,038	$927,085,485	5.1	0.28

(Continued)

	1	2	3	4	5
				Average Length of Stay	
			Medicare	of Stay	Cost to
DRG^A	Diagnosis	Covered Charges	Reimbursement	(Days)	Charge
321	MED KIDNEY & URINARY TRACT INFECTIONS AGE > 17 W/O	$314,743,801	$77,649,965	3.6	0.25
322	MED KIDNEY & URINARY TRACT INFECTIONS AGE 0–17	$880,694	$180,291	3.6	0.20
323	MED URINARY STONES W CC, &/OR ESW LITHOTRIPSY	$294,180,676	$75,605,954	3.1	0.26
324	MED URINARY STONES W/O CC	$46,569,583	$9,532,728	1.9	0.20
325	MED KIDNEY & URINARY TRACT SIGNS & SYMPTOMS AGE > 17	$111,638,765	$31,139,960	3.7	0.28
326	MED KIDNEY & URINARY TRACT SIGNS & SYMPTOMS AGE > 17	$20,833,330	$4,820,528	2.6	0.23
327	MED KIDNEY & URINARY TRACT SIGNS & SYMPTOMS AGE 0–17	—	—	—	—
328	MED URETHRAL STRICTURE AGE > 17 W CC	$7,845,831	$2,269,949	3.5	0.29
329	MED URETHRAL STRICTURE AGE > 17 W/O CC	$685,218	$195,272	2	0.28
330	MED URETHRAL STRICTURE AGE 0–17	—	—	—	—
331	MED OTHER KIDNEY & URINARY TRACT DIAGNOSES AGE > 17	$1,066,134,143	$315,716,185	5.4	0.30
332	MED OTHER KIDNEY & URINARY TRACT DIAGNOSES AGE > 17	$51,048,930	$12,977,533	3.1	0.25

	1	2	3	4	5
DRG[A]	**Diagnosis**	**Covered Charges**	**Medicare Reimbursement**	**Average Length of Stay (Days)**	**Cost to Charge**
333	MED OTHER KIDNEY & URINARY TRACT DIAGNOSES AGE 0–17	$6,768,922	$1,868,428	5.5	0.28
334	SURG MAJOR MALE PELVIC PROCEDURES W CC	$258,628,599	$72,640,529	4.3	0.28
335	SURG MAJOR MALE PELVIC PROCEDURES W/O CC	$244,702,790	$61,009,339	2.7	0.25
336	SURG TRANSURETHRAL PROSTATECTOMY W CC	$462,377,580	$126,226,818	3.3	0.27
337	SURG TRANSURETHRAL PROSTATECTOMY W/O CC	$252,578,607	$60,426,161	1.9	0.24
338	SURG TESTES PROCEDURES, FOR MALIGNANCY	$16,426,887	$4,047,291	6.2	0.25
339	SURG TESTES PROCEDURES, NON-MALIGNANCY AGE > 17	$26,871,011	$7,696,259	5.1	0.29
340	SURG TESTES PROCEDURES, NON-MALIGNANCY AGE 0–17	—	—	—	—
341	SURG PENIS PROCEDURES	$73,960,021	$21,873,907	3.2	0.30
342	SURG CIRCUMCISION AGE > 17	$8,593,169	$1,992,371	3.4	0.23
343	SURG CIRCUMCISION AGE 0–17	—	—	—	—

(Continued)

	1	2	3	4	5
				Average Length of Stay	
			Medicare	of Stay	Cost to
DRG^A	Diagnosis	Covered Charges	Reimbursement	(Days)	Charge
344	SURG OTHER MALE REPRODUCTIVE SYSTEM O.R. PROCEDUR	$60,752,850	$18,605,763	2.7	0.31
345	SURG OTHER MALE REPRODUCTIVE SYSTEM O.R. PROC EXC	$30,650,554	$9,220,059	4.8	0.30
346	MED MALIGNANCY, MALE REPRODUCTIVE SYSTEM, W CC	$76,945,526	$21,613,196	5.7	0.28
347	MED MALIGNANCY, MALE REPRODUCTIVE SYSTEM, W/O CC	$2,937,849	$640,066	3.1	0.22
348	MED BENIGN PROSTATIC HYPERTROPHY W CC	$54,147,648	$15,047,213	4.1	0.28
349	MED BENIGN PROSTATIC HYPERTROPHY W/O CC	$4,447,367	$1,158,386	2.4	0.26
350	MED INFLAMMATION OF THE MALE REPRODUCTIVE SYSTEM	$92,815,120	$24,465,021	4.5	0.26
351	MED STERILIZATION, MALE	—	—	—	—
352	MED OTHER MALE REPRODUCTIVE SYSTEM DIAGNOSES	$13,160,877	$3,498,234	4	0.27
353	SURG PELVIC EVISCERATION, RADICAL HYSTERECTOMY &	$107,131,989	$31,453,418	6.3	0.29
354	SURG UTERINE, ADNEXA PROC FOR NON-OVARIAN/ADNEXAL	$221,934,647	$65,132,216	5.7	0.29

	1	**2**	**3**	**4**	**5**
DRG[A]	**Diagnosis**	**Covered Charges**	**Medicare Reimbursement**	**Average Length of Stay (Days)**	**Cost to Charge**
355	SURG UTERINE, ADN-EXA PROC FOR NON-OVARIAN/ADNEXAL	$81,321,616	$21,570,007	3.1	0.27
356	SURG FEMALE REPRODUCTIVE SYSTEM RECON-STRUCTIVE PR	$308,329,724	$76,276,762	1.9	0.25
357	SURG UTERINE & ADNEXA PROC FOR OVARIAN OR ADNEXAL	$235,167,958	$75,494,387	8.1	0.32
358	SURG UTERINE & ADNEXA PROC FOR NON-MALIGNANCY W C	$428,506,407	$120,079,369	4	0.28
359	SURG UTERINE & ADNEXA PROC FOR NON-MALIGNANCY W/O	$401,711,476	$98,948,327	2.4	0.25
360	SURG VAGINA, CERVIX & VULVA PROCEDURES	$226,654,509	$58,930,553	2.6	0.26
361	SURG LAPAROSCOPY & INCISIONAL TUBAL INTERRUPTION	$5,498,157	$1,417,812	3	0.26
362	SURG ENDOSCOPIC TUBAL INTERRUPTION	—	—	—	—
363	SURG D&C, CONIZATION & RADIO-IMPLANT, FOR MALIGNA	$40,288,470	$11,065,856	3.8	0.27
364	SURG D&C, CONIZA-TION EXCEPT FOR MALIGNANCY	$23,277,524	$6,738,935	4.2	0.29

(Continued)

	1	2	3	4	5
				Average Length of Stay	
			Medicare	of Stay	Cost to
DRG[A]	Diagnosis	Covered Charges	Reimbursement	(Days)	Charge
365	SURG OTHER FEMALE REPRODUCTIVE SYSTEM O.R. PROCED	$61,131,474	$20,190,553	7.7	0.33
366	MED MALIGNANCY, FEMALE REPRODUCTIVE SYSTEM W CC	$111,090,686	$34,851,497	6.6	0.31
367	MED MALIGNANCY, FEMALE REPRODUCTIVE SYSTEM W/O CC	$5,256,495	$1,398,612	3.1	0.27
368	MED INFECTIONS, FEMALE REPRODUCTIVE SYSTEM	$84,943,495	$24,511,796	6.7	0.29
369	MED MENSTRUAL & OTHER FEMALE REPRODUCTIVE SYSTEM	$43,248,553	$11,089,853	3.3	0.26
370	SURG CESAREAN SECTION W CC	$33,281,841	$10,447,636	5.2	0.31
371	SURG CESAREAN SECTION W/O CC	$25,933,550	$6,315,724	3.4	0.24
372	MED VAGINAL DELIVERY W COMPLICATING DIAGNOSES	$11,591,954	$3,199,657	3.2	0.28
373	MED VAGINAL DELIVERY W/O COMPLICATING DIAGNOSES	$33,244,861	$7,298,133	2.2	0.22
374	SURG VAGINAL DELIVERY W STERILIZATION &/OR D&C	$1,856,909	$534,350	2.8	0.29
375	SURG VAGINAL DELIVERY W O.R. PROC EXCEPT STERIL &	—	—	—	—

	1	2	3	4	5
				Average Length	
			Medicare	**of Stay**	**Cost to**
DRG^A	**Diagnosis**	**Covered Charges**	**Reimbursement**	**(Days)**	**Charge**
376	MED POSTPARTUM & POST ABORTION DIAGNOSES W/O O.R.	$5,300,048	$1,720,547	4.3	0.32
377	SURG POSTPARTUM & POST ABORTION DIAGNOSES W O.R.	$2,697,811	$659,594	4.5	0.24
378	MED ECTOPIC PREGNANCY	$2,813,149	$779,791	2.3	0.28
379	MED THREATENED ABORTION	$3,676,075	$840,902	2.9	0.23
380	MED ABORTION W/O D&C	$590,699	$157,187	2.1	0.27
381	SURG ABORTION W D&C, ASPIRATION CURETTAGE OR HYST	$2,500,529	$552,488	2.3	0.22
382	MED FALSE LABOR	$184,861	$32,690	1.5	0.18
383	MED OTHER ANTEPAR-TUM DIAGNOSES W MEDICAL COMPLICA	$28,410,817	$7,971,425	4.2	0.28
384	MED OTHER ANTEPAR-TUM DIAGNOSES W/O MEDICAL COMPLI	$885,054	$204,290	2.6	0.23
385	MED NEONATES, DIED OR TRANSFERRED TO ANOTHER ACU	—	—	—	—
386	MED EXTREME IMMA-TURITY OR RESPIRA-TORY DISTRESS S	—	—	—	—
387	MED PREMATURITY W MAJOR PROBLEMS	—	—	—	—
388	MED PREMATU-RITY W/O MAJOR PROBLEMS	—	—	—	—

(Continued)

	1	2	3	4	5
DRG[A]	**Diagnosis**	**Covered Charges**	**Medicare Reimbursement**	**Average Length of Stay (Days)**	**Cost to Charge**
389	MED FULL TERM NEONATE W MAJOR PROBLEMS	—	—	—	—
390	MED NEONATE W OTHER SIGNIFICANT PROBLEMS	—	—	—	—
391	MED NORMAL NEWBORN	—	—	—	—
392	6 SURG SPLENEC-TOMY AGE > 17	$121,196,273	$42,388,588	9.2	0.35
393	6 SURG SPLENEC-TOMY AGE 0–17	—	—	—	—
394	6 SURG OTHER O.R. PROCEDURES OF THE BLOOD AND BLOOD	$100,295,058	$31,509,949	7.4	0.31
395	6 MED RED BLOOD CELL DISORDERS AGE > 17	$1,692,467,984	$467,769,995	4.3	0.28
396	6 MED RED BLOOD CELL DISORDERS AGE 0–17	—	—	—	—
397	6 MED COAGULATION DISORDERS	$472,813,259	$152,036,296	5.2	0.32
398	6 MED RETICU-LOENDOTHELIAL & IMMUNITY DISORDERS W CC	$416,003,799	$126,660,347	5.7	0.30
399	6 MED RETICULOEN-DOTHELIAL & IMMU-NITY DISORDERS W/O	$19,959,677	$5,223,476	3.3	0.26
400	SURG NO LONGER VALID	—	—	—	—

DRG^A	Diagnosis	1 Covered Charges	2 Medicare Reimbursement	3 Average Length of Stay (Days)	4	5 Cost to Charge

DRG^A	Diagnosis	Covered Charges	Medicare Reimbursement	Average Length of Stay (Days)	Cost to Charge
401	SURG LYMPHOMA & NON-ACUTE LEUKE-MIA W OTHER O.R. P	$342,426,863	$109,438,188	11	0.32
402	SURG LYMPHOMA & NON-ACUTE LEUKE-MIA W OTHER O.R. P	$31,032,388	$8,431,432	4	0.27
403	MED LYMPHOMA & NON-ACUTE LEUKE-MIA W CC	$1,077,876,490	$340,921,003	8	0.32
404	MED LYMPHOMA & NON-ACUTE LEUKE-MIA W/O CC	$68,620,205	$18,578,429	4.2	0.27
405	MED ACUTE LEUKE-MIA W/O MAJOR O.R. PROCEDURE AGE 0–17	—	—	—	—
406	SURG MYELOPROLIF DISORD OR POORLY DIFF NEOPL W MA	$121,527,586	$37,662,945	9.8	0.31
407	SURG MYELOPROLIF DISORD OR POORLY DIFF NEOPL W MA	$15,193,798	$4,219,596	4	0.28
408	SURG MYELOPROLIF DISORD OR POORLY DIFF NEOPL W OT	$94,620,256	$30,348,546	8.1	0.32
409	MED RADIOTHERAPY	$43,819,845	$14,097,061	5.8	0.32
410	MED CHEMOTHERAPY W/O ACUTE LEUKE-MIA AS SECONDARY	$637,239,163	$196,553,689	3.9	0.31
411	MED HISTORY OF MALIGNANCY W/O ENDOSCOPY	$102,976	$31,440	3.3	0.31
412	MED HISTORY OF MALIGNANCY W ENDOSCOPY	$187,396	$35,009	2.6	0.19

(Continued)

	1	2	3	4	5
DRG[A]	Diagnosis	Covered Charges	Medicare Reimbursement	Average Length of Stay (Days)	Cost to Charge
413	MED OTHER MYELO-PROLIF DIS OR POORLY DIFF NEOPL DI	$122,783,906	$36,992,233	6.8	0.30
414	MED OTHER MYELO-PROLIF DIS OR POORLY DIFF NEOPL DI	$8,727,605	$2,182,583	4	0.25
415	SURG O.R. PROCE-DURE FOR INFECTIOUS & PARASITIC DI	$3,442,535,294	$1,121,588,164	14.1	0.33
416	MED SEPTICEMIA AGE > 17	$7,028,011,768	$2,049,454,882	7.4	0.29
417	MED SEPTICEMIA AGE 0–17	$388,603	$134,715	3.9	0.35
418	MED POSTOPERATIVE & POST-TRAUMATIC INFECTIONS	$560,377,399	$172,094,754	6.2	0.31
419	MED FEVER OF UNKNOWN ORIGIN AGE > 17 W CC	$250,048,310	$70,023,066	4.4	0.28
420	MED FEVER OF UNKNOWN ORIGIN AGE > 17 W/O CC	$32,197,903	$8,401,261	3.4	0.26
421	MED VIRAL ILLNESS AGE > 17	$164,010,440	$42,226,294	4.1	0.26
422	MED VIRAL ILLNESS & FEVER OF UNKNOWN ORIGIN AGE	$775,108	$243,189	3.7	0.31
423	MED OTHER INFEC-TIOUS & PARASITIC DISEASES DIAGNOS	$304,225,281	$91,813,125	8.3	0.30
424	SURG O.R. PROCE-DURE W PRINCIPAL DIAGNOSES OF MENT	$83,682,807	$27,194,764	15.6	0.32

| | **1** | **2** | **3** | **4**
Average
Length
of Stay | **5** |
DRG^A	Diagnosis	Covered Charges	Medicare Reimbursement	(Days)	Cost to Charge
425	MED ACUTE ADJUST- MENT REACTION & PSYCHOSOCIAL DYSF	$215,281,914	$69,000,143	4.5	0.32
426	MED DEPRESSIVE NEUROSES	$188,738,212	$68,090,102	6.3	0.36
427	MED NEUROSES EX- CEPT DEPRESSIVE	$53,724,247	$20,082,405	5.7	0.37
428	MED DISORDERS OF PERSONALITY & IMPULSE CONTROL	$41,249,032	$15,378,991	9.1	0.37
429	MED ORGANIC DIS- TURBANCES & MEN- TAL RETARDATION	$999,817,047	$385,362,893	9.3	0.39
430	MED PSYCHOSES	$5,791,463,398	$2,122,548,692	10.7	0.37
431	MED CHILDHOOD MENTAL DISORDERS	$21,721,510	$7,598,698	9.3	0.35
432	MED OTHER MENTAL DISORDER DIAGNOSES	$6,378,492	$2,104,115	5.1	0.33
433	MED ALCOHOL/DRUG ABUSE OR DEPEND- ENCE, LEFT AMA	$32,612,087	$8,503,900	3	0.26
434	MED NO LONGER VALID	—	—	—	—
435	MED NO LONGER VALID	—	—	—	—
436	MED NO LONGER VALID	—	—	—	—
437	MED NO LONGER VALID	—	—	—	—
438	NO LONGER VALID	—	—	—	—
439	SURG SKIN GRAFTS FOR INJURIES	$64,321,958	$19,334,031	8.9	0.30

(Continued)

DRG[A]	Diagnosis	1 Covered Charges	2 Medicare Reimbursement	3 Average Length of Stay (Days)	4 Cost to Charge	5

DRG[A]	Diagnosis	Covered Charges	Medicare Reimbursement	Average Length of Stay (Days)	Cost to Charge
440	SURG WOUND DEBRIDEMENTS FOR INJURIES	$190,739,221	$63,123,400	8.8	0.33
441	SURG HAND PROCE- DURES FOR INJURIES	$13,690,569	$3,662,330	3.4	0.27
442	SURG OTHER O.R. PROCEDURES FOR INJURIES W CC	$825,322,601	$261,022,064	8.7	0.32
443	SURG OTHER O.R. PROCEDURES FOR INJURIES W/O CC	$61,257,286	$16,881,771	3.4	0.28
444	MED TRAUMATIC IN- JURY AGE > 17 W CC	$80,130,407	$21,152,389	4.1	0.26
445	MED TRAUMATIC INJU- RY AGE > 17 W/O CC	$21,663,714	$4,960,035	2.9	0.23
446	MED TRAUMATIC INJURY AGE 0–17	—	—	—	—
447	MED ALLERGIC REAC- TIONS AGE > 17	$64,481,183	$14,765,553	2.6	0.23
448	MED ALLERGIC REAC- TIONS AGE 0–17	—	—	—	—
449	MED POISONING & TOXIC EFFECTS OF DRUGS AGE > 17 W	$610,936,749	$168,328,594	3.7	0.28
450	MED POISONING & TOXIC EFFECTS OF DRUGS AGE > 17 W	$60,620,169	$13,720,852	2	0.23
451	MED POISONING & TOXIC EFFECTS OF DRUGS AGE 0–17	—	—	—	—
452	MED COMPLICATIONS OF TREATMENT W CC	$537,419,642	$161,873,903	4.9	0.30

	1	2	3	4	5
				Average Length	
			Medicare	of Stay	Cost to
DRG^A	Diagnosis	Covered Charges	Reimbursement	(Days)	Charge
453	MED COMPLICATIONS OF TREATMENT W/O CC	$53,071,567	$13,634,011	2.8	0.26
454	MED OTHER INJURY, POISONING & TOXIC EFFECT DIAG W	$57,576,652	$15,809,363	4.1	0.27
455	MED OTHER INJURY, POISONING & TOXIC EFFECT DIAG W	$7,776,424	$1,791,261	2.2	0.23
456	NO LONGER VALID	—	—	—	—
457	MED NO LONGER VALID	—	—	—	—
458	SURG NO LONGER VALID	—	—	—	—
459	SURG NO LONGER VALID	—	—	—	—
460	MED NO LONGER VALID	—	—	—	—
461	SURG O.R. PROC W DIAGNOSES OF OTHER CONTACT W HEA	$273,361,492	$91,902,046	12.8	0.34
462	MED REHABILITATION	$7,438,494,878	$3,919,264,650	11.7	0.53
463	MED SIGNS & SYMPTOMS W CC	$395,045,016	$111,819,242	4.1	0.28
464	MED SIGNS & SYMPTOMS W/O CC	$70,258,957	$17,722,305	3	0.25
465	MED AFTERCARE W HISTORY OF MALIGNANCY AS SECONDAR	$3,991,579	$1,502,350	5.1	0.38
466	MED AFTERCARE W/O HISTORY OF MALIGNANCY AS SECOND	$25,925,757	$9,495,708	5.9	0.37

(Continued)

DRG^A	Diagnosis	1 Covered Charges	2 Medicare Reimbursement	3 Average Length of Stay (Days)	4 Cost to Charge 5
467	MED OTHER FACTORS INFLUENCING HEALTH STATUS	$11,469,494	$3,908,817	3.4	0.34
468	XTENSIVE O.R. PROCE-DURE UNRELATED TO PRINCIPAL DIAG	$3,675,824,235	$1,149,788,909	12.7	0.31
469	* PRINCIPAL DIAG-NOSIS INVALID AS DISCHARGE DIAGNOSI	—	—	—	—
470	* UNGROUPABLE	—	—	—	—
471	SURG BILATERAL OR MULTIPLE MAJOR JOINT PROCS OF LO	$828,794,309	$248,125,238	5.1	0.30
472	SURG NO LONGER VALID	—	—	—	—
473	MED ACUTE LEUKE-MIA W/O MAJOR O.R. PROCEDURE AGE >	$588,246,446	$206,654,882	12.7	0.35
474	SURG NO LONGER VALID	—	—	—	—
475	MED RESPIRATORY SYSTEM DIAGNOSIS WITH VENTILATOR S	$7,374,038,076	$2,385,817,254	11	0.32
476	URG PROSTATIC O.R. PROCEDURE UNRE-LATED TO PRINCIPAL	$125,864,152	$39,336,642	10.5	0.31
477	URG NON-EXTENSIVE O.R. PROCEDURE UNRELATED TO PRINC	$887,739,255	$267,697,618	8.2	0.30
478	SURG OTHER VAS-CULAR PROCEDURES W CC	$4,927,298,075	$1,514,102,382	7.1	0.31

	1	2	3	4	5
				Average Length of Stay	Cost to
DRG[A]	Diagnosis	Covered Charges	Medicare Reimbursement	(Days)	Charge
479	SURG OTHER VAS-CULAR PROCEDURES W/O CC	$629,481,884	$177,038,815	2.8	0.28
480	RE SURG LIVER TRANSPLANT	$282,720,653	$87,651,006	17.2	0.31
481	RE SURG BONE MAR-ROW TRANSPLANT	$176,718,360	$57,791,910	21.9	0.33
482	RE SURG TRACHE-OSTOMY FOR FACE, MOUTH & NECK DIAGNOSE	$331,334,059	$118,257,059	11.4	0.36
483	RE SURG TRAC W MECH VENT 6+HRS OR PDX EXCEPT FACE,	$13,117,170,169	$4,569,858,033	37.8	0.35
484	SURG CRANIOTOMY FOR MULTIPLE SIGNIFI-CANT TRAUMA	$48,094,700	$15,710,134	12.8	0.33
485	SURG LIMB REAT-TACHMENT, HIP AND FEMUR PROC FOR MU	$207,452,972	$64,338,239	9.7	0.31
486	SURG OTHER O.R. PROCEDURES FOR MULTIPLE SIGNIFICA	$256,198,239	$80,872,216	12.4	0.32
487	MED OTHER MULTIPLE SIGNIFICANT TRAUMA	$173,388,077	$50,920,333	7.2	0.29
488	SURG HIV W EXTEN-SIVE O.R. PROCEDURE	$77,256,540	$26,873,733	16.3	0.35
489	MED HIV W MAJOR RELATED CONDITION	$509,903,402	$173,433,643	8.4	0.34
490	MED HIV W OR W/O OTHER RELATED CONDITION	$115,317,740	$35,055,191	5.4	0.30

(Continued)

	1	2	3	4	5
				Average Length	
			Medicare	of Stay	Cost to
DRG[A]	Diagnosis	Covered Charges	Reimbursement	(Days)	Charge
491	SURG MAJOR JOINT & LIMB REATTACHMENT PROCEDURES OF	$581,909,273	$169,420,493	3.1	0.29
492	MED CHEMOTHERAPY W ACUTE LEUKEMIA OR W USE OF HI	$312,939,956	$112,570,458	13.6	0.36
493	SURG LAPAROSCOPIC CHOLECYSTECTOMY W/O C.D.E. W CC	$1,946,520,371	$567,945,521	6.1	0.29
494	SURG LAPAROSCOPIC CHOLECYSTECTOMY W/O C.D.E. W/O C	$452,643,390	$116,550,407	2.7	0.26
495	RE SURG LUNG TRANSPLANT	$84,851,808	$23,324,369	16.9	0.27
496	SURG COMBINED ANTERIOR/POSTERIOR SPINAL FUSION	$683,635,516	$239,401,123	6.4	0.35
497	SURG SPINAL FUSION EXCEPT CERVICAL W CC	$1,708,244,668	$500,912,025	6	0.29
498	SURG SPINAL FUSION EXCEPT CERVICAL W/O CC	$832,279,951	$224,736,767	3.8	0.27
499	SURG BACK & NECK PROCEDURES EXCEPT SPINAL FUSION W	$888,265,440	$256,188,554	4.3	0.29
500	SURG BACK & NECK PROCEDURES EXCEPT SPINAL FUSION W	$782,804,487	$205,334,082	2.2	0.26
501	SURG KNEE PROCE- DURES W PDX OF INFECTION W CC	$136,980,571	$44,729,001	9.9	0.33

	1	2	3	4	5
DRG[A]	Diagnosis	Covered Charges	Medicare Reimbursement	Average Length of Stay (Days)	Cost to Charge
502	SURG KNEE PROCE-DURES W PDX OF INFECTION W/O CC	$17,951,537	$5,143,338	5.7	0.29
503	SURG KNEE PROCE-DURES W/O PDX OF INFECTION	$126,551,717	$35,511,302	3.8	0.28
504	SURG EXTENSIVE RD DEGREE BURNS W SKIN GRAFT	$37,179,678	$13,617,441	27.5	0.37
505	MED EXTENSIVE RD DEGREE BURNS W/O SKIN GRAFT	$4,854,837	$2,263,141	3	0.47
506	SURG FULL THICKNESS BURN W SKIN GRAFT OR INHAL IN	$107,975,580	$35,767,091	16.7	0.33
507	SURG FULL THICKNESS BURN W SKIN GRFT OR INHAL INJ	$11,590,902	$3,707,740	8.6	0.32
508	MED FULL THICKNESS BURN W/O SKIN GRFT OR INHAL IN	$16,674,829	$5,539,234	7.4	0.33
509	MED FULL THICKNESS BURN W/O SKIN GRFT OR INH INJ	$2,919,660	$618,848	5.2	0.21
510	MED NON-EXTENSIVE BURNS W CC OR SIGNIFICANT TRAUM	$46,006,301	$14,241,624	6.6	0.31
511	MED NON-EXTENSIVE BURNS W/O CC OR SIGNIFICANT TRA	$10,348,589	$2,981,466	4.1	0.29
512	RE SURG SIMULTANE-OUS PANCREAS/ KIDNEY TRANSPLANT	$109,654,957	$18,746,820	12.8	0.17

(Continued)

	1	2	3	4	5
				Average Length	
			Medicare	of Stay	Cost to
DRG[A]	Diagnosis	Covered Charges	Reimbursement	(Days)	Charge
513	RE SURG PANCREAS TRANSPLANT	$30,290,082	$8,950,180	10	0.30
514	SURG NO LONGER VALID	—	—	—	—
515	SURG CARDIAC DEFI-BRILLATOR IMPLANT W/O CARDIAC CAT	$2,681,002,072	$829,424,925	4.3	0.31
516	SURG PERCUTANEOUS CARDIOVASC PROC W AMI	$1,751,339,390	$539,360,112	4.8	0.31
517	SURG PERC CARDIO PROC W NON-DRUG ELUTING STENT W/O	$2,372,140,790	$721,136,493	2.6	0.30
518	SURG PERC CARDIO PROC W/O CORONARY ARTERY STENT OR	$1,348,970,933	$390,372,826	3.5	0.29
519	SURG CERVICAL SPI-NAL FUSION W CC	$519,836,772	$149,925,531	4.8	0.29
520	SURG CERVICAL SPI-NAL FUSION W/O CC	$457,019,573	$115,436,646	2	0.25
521	0 MED ALCOHOL/DRUG ABUSE OR DEPENDENCE W CC	$480,542,289	$146,933,451	5.8	0.31
522	0 MED ALC/DRUG ABUSE OR DEPEND W REHABILITATION THE	$61,744,207	$19,561,299	9.5	0.32
523	0 MED ALC/DRUG ABUSE OR DEPEND W/O REHABILITATION T	$167,932,248	$50,967,395	4.4	0.30
524	MED TRANSIENT ISCHEMIA	$1,522,594,261	$390,052,924	3.2	0.26
525	SURG HEART ASSIST SYSTEM IMPLANT	$122,734,967	$38,979,209	25.4	0.32

	1	2	3	4	5
				Average Length	
			Medicare	of Stay	Cost to
DRG^A	Diagnosis	Covered Charges	Reimbursement	(Days)	Charge
526	SURG PERCUTNE-OUS CARDIOVASU-LAR PROC W DRUG ELUTING	$2,957,710,449	$895,170,665	4.4	0.30
527	SURG PERCUTNE-OUS CARDIOVASU-LAR PROC W DRUG ELUTING	$7,984,503,371	$2,466,431,823	2.2	0.31
528	SURG INTRACRANIAL VASCULAR PROC W PDX HEMORRHAGE	$258,280,313	$86,026,626	17.2	0.33
529	SURG VENTRICULAR SHUNT PROCEDURES W CC	$172,162,063	$55,920,272	8	0.32
530	SURG VENTRICULAR SHUNT PROCEDURES W/O CC	$52,741,751	$15,245,372	3.1	0.29
531	SURG SPINAL PROCE-DURES W CC	$280,317,531	$88,682,663	9.4	0.32
532	SURG SPINAL PROCE-DURES W/O CC	$71,650,909	$20,033,187	3.7	0.28
533	SURG EXTRACRANIAL PROCEDURES W CC	$1,311,827,706	$402,498,779	3.8	0.31
534	SURG EXTRACRANIAL PROCEDURES W/O CC	$803,262,242	$227,139,334	1.8	0.28
535	SURG CARDIAC DEFIB IMPLANT W CARDIAC CATH W AMI/HF	$1,732,118,797	$608,492,646	8.3	0.35
536	SURG CARDIAC DEFIB IMPLANT W CARDIAC CATH W/O AMI/	$2,164,512,327	$695,171,767	5.4	0.32
537	SURG LOCAL EXCIS & REMOV OF INT FIX DEV EXCEPT HIP	$284,040,897	$86,669,380	6.8	0.31

(Continued)

	1	2	3	4	5
				Average Length of Stay	
			Medicare	of Stay	Cost to
DRG[A]	Diagnosis	Covered Charges	Reimbursement	(Days)	Charge
538	SURG LOCAL EXCIS & REMOV OF INT FIX DEV EXCEPT HIP	$100,012,928	$26,598,457	2.8	0.27
539	7 SURG LYMPHOMA & LEUKEMIA W MAJOR OR PROCEDURE W C	$311,793,279	$106,392,954	10.7	0.34
540	7 SURG LYMPHOMA & LEUKEMIA W MAJOR OR PROCEDURE W/O	$35,523,450	$11,106,815	3.6	0.31
TOTAL		$332,991,884,450	$101,335,003,733	5.8	0.30

[A]Short-stay inpatient diagnosis-related groups.

GLOSSARY

Abridged life table. A means for converting mortality rates into the average life expectancy of a hypothetical cohort of 100,000 persons exposed to the mortality rates. In an abridged life table, mortality rates in n-year intervals are used to estimate the expected number of deaths in a hypothetical cohort of 100,000 persons. From these deaths, the mean number of years lived by the cohort is calculated. Although abridged life tables use larger age intervals than standard life tables, the two methods produce similar results as long as the interval is reasonably short.

Accuracy. The extent to which a measured value is representative of its real value.

Analytical horizon. The period over which all costs and outcomes are considered in an economic analysis.

Appropriate technology utilization. The prioritization of the most cost-effective technologies over less cost-effective technologies (for example, vaccination versus heart-lung transplants).

Attribute. A given measure of health. For instance, pain on a 1 to 5 scale is a health attribute.

Baseline value. The most likely value of an uncertain parameter.

Bias. A form of nonrandom error in which some force acts to systematically influence the measurement of a given value such that it deviates from its true value. For instance, when men are asked their height, they tend to overestimate values measured by a third party.

Charge. The amount billed by a given provider, including profits. A charge is almost invariably greater than the opportunity cost of the services provided.

Clinical practice guidelines. A standardized practice algorithm for diagnosing and treating disease that has been designed with the input of experts.

Community-derived preferences. Preferences for health states derived from a general population rather than from persons with the disease of interest.

Competing alternative. An alternative practice for diagnosing or treating the disease you are studying in your cost-effectiveness analysis. For instance, the competing alternative for annual screening mammography might be monthly breast self-examination.

Cost-effectiveness analysis. A type of economic analysis in which costs associated with two or more strategies are compared based on some measure of effectiveness. In health, cost-effectiveness and cost utility are often used interchangeably.

Cost-to-charge ratio. A ratio used to convert medical charges to something more representative of their societal opportunity cost.

Cost-utility analysis. A type of economic analysis that compares the costs associated with two or more strategies based on a measure of utility. In the reference case analysis, the measure of utility must be a quality-adjusted life year–compatible health-related quality of life score.

Cross-sectional studies. Studies that contain observational data at a single point in time. For instance, a census is a cross-sectional study of the characteristics of the general population of a country.

Crude rates. Rates unadjusted for age, gender, or other sociodemographic characteristics.

Data extraction tool. Software that allows users to easily obtain values from a given dataset.

Decision analysis model. A model used to calculate the expected value of a given health strategy. Decision analysis models are the most frequently used means for calculating incremental cost-effectiveness ratios.

Dimension. A given measure of health—for instance, pain on a 1 to 5 scale is a dimension of health.

Direct costs. Costs associated with goods and services consumed, such as units of influenza vaccine used in a vaccination drive.

Discounting. The process of converting future costs into present terms. The rate of discount used in cost-effectiveness analysis is 3 percent for both costs and quality-adjusted life years.

Domain. A given measure of health—for instance, pain on a 1 to 5 scale is a health domain.

Dominant strategy. A strategy that is more effective and less expensive than at least one competing alternative.

Dominated strategy. A strategy that is less effective and more costly than at least one competing alternative.

Double-blinded. An experimental study design in which neither the subject nor the investigator is aware of the treatment administered to a subject.

Effectiveness. The performance of health interventions in the real world.

Effect size. The strength of the relationship between two variables.

Efficacy. The performance of health interventions under exacting laboratory conditions.

Expected value. The probabilistically weighted average of a series of numbers.

Expenditure. The amount of money paid for a service.

External validity. The extent to which the results of a study are generalizable to settings other than the one in which the data were collected.

False-positive test result. A false-positive test result occurs when a laboratory test indicates that disease is present when in fact it is absent.

Fixed costs. Costs that do not change when a health intervention is applied.

Governmental perspective. An analysis that includes costs and effectiveness benefits from the perspective of only a governmental agency. For instance, such analysis includes the cost of treatments paid for by the government but not costs incurred by patients.

Gross cost. An aggregate cost associated with a health event. For instance, the cost of hospitalization for influenza might be obtained from billing records. Such costs typically include most, but not all, products and services delivered for the particular health event.

Gross costing. The process of obtaining gross costs, usually from an electronic dataset.

Health intervention. A strategy for diagnosing or treating a disease.

Health outcome. *See* Outcome, health.

Health-related quality of life (HRQL) score. A numerical valuation of life in a given health state anchored between 0 (death) and 1 (perfect health). These scores are used to adjust life years to quality-adjusted life years (QALYs). Thus, a year of life lived at an HRQL of 0.7 is equivalent to 0.7 QALYs (or 0.7 years of perfect health).

Health state. The health status of a given person or population at one point in time. Examples are hospitalized, ill, alive, well, and dead.

Health status. The overall state of health of an individual or group of individuals. Health status can also be defined as the sum of various health states.

Healthy volunteer effect. Subjects who volunteer for a study are typically healthier than the average person residing in the community from which the subjects were recruited. Because healthy people are not representative of the population at large, the results of studies using such subjects may be biased.

Hypothetical cohort. A study cohort derived from statistical data rather than an actual cohort of subjects. For instance, life tables are constructed based on hypothetical numbers of deaths occurring among a group of 100,000 hypothetical subjects exposed to real-world age-specific mortality rates.

Incidence rate. Number of new cases over a given time interval divided by the population at risk over the same interval.

Incremental value. A cost or effectiveness value above and beyond the average value. For instance, if a woman receiving annual mammography can expect to live eleven years and a woman who does not receive mammography can expect to live ten years, the incremental gain in life expectancy is 11 years − 10 years = 1 year.

Indirect costs. Costs not directly related to the consumption of goods or services. Lost productivity due to illness is an example of an indirect cost.

Intangible costs. Costs for which it is difficult to attach a monetary value.

League table. A table of interventions listed by their incremental cost-effectiveness ratios. If the incremental cost-effectiveness ratios for most interventions are known, a league table can theoretically be used to maximize the number of lives saved within a given health budget.

Leisure time costs. The monetary valuation of time away from work. In cost-effectiveness analysis, leisure time costs are typically thought of as the time during which persons cannot enjoy the time spent away from work because they are ill.

Levels of evidence. A method used to rank the appropriateness of studies based on their research design.

Longitudinal studies. *See* Prospective studies.

Lost productivity costs. Costs associated with the time a person cannot work. In cost-effectiveness analysis, lost productivity is typically measured as time lost due to illness.

Marginal value. A cost or effectiveness value above and beyond the baseline measure. For instance, if a woman receiving annual mammography can expect to live eleven years and a woman who does not receive mammography can expect to live ten years, the marginal gain in life expectancy is 11 years − 10 years = 1 year. Typically, the term *incremental* is preferred in cost-effectiveness analysis.

Markov model. A decision analysis model that incorporates an element of time.

Medical Expenditure Panel Survey (MEPS). An annual survey of around 40,000 households in the United States. It includes a household component with demographic and health information of the participants. It also contains a provider component that obtains the cost of medical visits from providers. This is the most important dataset for cost-effectiveness analysis available in the United States.

Meta-analysis. An analytical form of literature review in which data from two or more individual studies are combined and reanalyzed as if they were a single study.

Micro cost. A cost obtained for a single product or service.

Micro-costing. The process of measuring, valuing, and then adding up the various cost components (goods or services) associated with a health event. For example, the cost of an influenza vaccination may include the cost of the vaccine itself, the cost of the syringe, and the time cost associated with administering the vaccine.

Misclassification bias. A form of nonrandom error associated with categorizing events. For instance, it is common for physicians to improperly categorize a patient's underlying cause of death in instances in which the patient suffered from multiple related diseases or conditions.

Monte Carlo simulation. A type of sensitivity analysis in which the range of values for each variable in a decision analysis model is assigned a probability distribution. Each distribution is then repeatedly sampled to obtain a mean and distribution for the overall value of interest (cost, effectiveness, or incremental cost-effectiveness).

Morbidity costs. The intangible costs associated with pain and suffering. In general economics, these costs are typically measured in terms of willingness-to-pay formulations. However, in cost-effectiveness analyses, they are measured in terms of changes in health-related quality of life.

Mortality cost. Costs related to human deaths. Some define these costs strictly in terms of the intangible value of human life lost, while others include tangible costs, such as burial costs, in this category.

Mortality rate. The number of deaths over a given time interval divided by the total number of people at risk of those deaths over that same time interval.

Multiattribute health status classification systems. Instruments used to generate preference scores.

Multiway sensitivity analysis. *See* Sensitivity analysis, multiway.

Net present value. The net value of future costs or returns discounted to present-day values.

Nonrandom error. *See* Bias.

Normal distribution. A probability distribution in which values are clustered toward the mean and then taper off, giving the distribution its characteristic bell-shaped curve. Also known as a bell curve or Gaussian distribution.

Odds ratios. A measure of effect size in which the odds of an event measured in one group are divided by the odds of the event occurring in another group. For instance, if the odds of death among those receiving a preventive intervention for diabetes is p and the odds of death among those who did not receive the treatment is q, then the odds ratio is $p(1 - q)/(1 - p)q$. The odds ratio is useful only when the outcome of interest is rare (occurs less than 5 percent of the time).

One-way sensitivity analysis. *See* Sensitivity analysis, one-way.

Opportunity cost. The value of the next best investment forgone.

Outcome, health. Any measure of health. Examples are diseases averted, life-years gained, and vaccine-preventable illnesses averted.

Piggyback study. A cost-effectiveness analysis conducted alongside a prospective cohort study.

Preference score. A weighted value for life lived with a given disease ranging from 0 to 1, where 0 represents death and 1 represents perfect health.

Preference-weighted generic instruments. An instrument used to generate health-related quality of life scores for various health states. The word *generic* indicates that the instrument is not typically applied to any disease in particular.

Prevalence. The number of people with a given disease.

Prevalence ratio. The number of people with a given disease divided by the total number of people at risk for that disease.

Prevalent cases. *See* Prevalence.

Primary cost-effectiveness analysis. A study, such as a randomized controlled trial, in which data are collected for the primary purpose of conducting a cost-effectiveness analysis.

Probability distribution. A series of values presented by the probability that they will be observed. For instance, a probability distribution of heights will have many values close to the mean and few values for people less than 3 feet (1 meter) tall or greater than 9 feet (3 meters) tall. As one approaches the mean, the probability of observing a given value increases.

Prospective studies. Studies in which subjects are followed over time. Typically this involves following subjects with and without putative risk factors for disease to ascertain who does and does not develop the disease.

QALY. *See* Quality-adjusted life year.

Quality-adjusted life expectancy (QALE). Life expectancy in perfect health. QALE is equal to the product of life expectancy and the age-adjusted health-related quality of life score.

Quality-adjusted life year (QALY). A year of life lived in perfect health.

Random error. Variance in a parameter estimate due to sampling error.

Randomized controlled trial. A form of experimental study in which subjects are randomly assigned to treatment conditions.

Recursive event. An event that repeats itself over time.

Reference case analysis. A standardized set of methods and theoretical frameworks for capturing costs, quality of life, and life expectancy in cost-effectiveness analysis. The reference case guidelines were forwarded by the Panel on Cost-Effectiveness in Health and Medicine.

Relative risk. *See* Risk ratio.

Reliable. An estimate that can be reproduced with relatively similar results from one study to the next.

Reproducible. *See* Reliable.

Retrospective studies. An experimental study design in which persons with an outcome of interest are compared to similar subjects who do not have the outcome of interest to ascertain whether a given exposure might have caused the outcome of interest.

Risk ratio. The ratio of the probability of an event occurring in an exposed group relative to the probability of the event's occurring in the unexposed group.

Robust analysis. An analysis in which one alternative remains dominant even after testing it over the high and low range of values in a sensitivity analysis.

Roll back. The term sometimes used when a decision analysis model is instructed to calculate the expected value of each strategy.

Sensitivity analysis. An analysis that varies model inputs over their plausible range of real-world value in order to examine how they might influence model outputs.

Sensitivity analysis, multiway. A test of the effect of error on model outputs in which three or more variables of interest are simultaneously varied over a range of plausible values while holding all other variables constant.

Sensitivity analysis, one-way. A test of the effect of error on model outputs in which the variable of interest is varied over a range of plausible values while holding all other variables constant.

Sensitivity analysis, tornado. A test of the effect of error on model outputs in which each variable of interest within the model is sequentially varied over a range of plausible values while holding all other variables constant. Graphs of the variables are stacked according to their overall influence on the model, so the output assumes the appearance of a tornado.

Sensitivity analysis, two-way. A test of the effect of error on model outputs in which two variables of interest are simultaneously varied over a range of plausible values while holding all other variables constant.

Simple decision analysis tree. A decision analysis tree that calculates the expected value of a series of probabilistically weighted events based on outcomes presented in present terms. This contrasts with a Markov model, which calculates changes in health states or costs from one year to the next.

Societal perspective. An analysis that includes all costs and benefits of a health intervention regardless of who is paying for it.

Standard deviation. A measure of the spread of a given set of numbers, calculated as the root mean squared deviation of these values from their mean.

Standard gamble. A method for calculating preference scores in which subjects are asked to trade life with a particular disease for a gamble between perfect health and death.

Standard life table. A means for converting mortality rates into the average life expectancy of a hypothetical cohort of 100,000 persons exposed to the mortality rates. In a standard life table, age-specific mortality rates in one-year intervals are used to estimate the expected number of deaths in a hypothetical cohort of 100,000 persons. From these deaths, the mean number of years lived by the cohort is calculated.

Standard of care. The best practice based on current scientific evidence.

State transition model. A decision analysis model that incorporates an element of time. Also known as a Markov model.

Statistical power. The likelihood that a statistical test will correctly identify a statistically significant difference between two means. In more technical terms, it is the probability that a test will reject a false null hypothesis.

Status quo. What is typically done in current medical practice. This can be a mix of treatments or diagnostic modalities.

Systematic bias. *See* Bias.

Threshold analysis. A one-way sensitivity analysis conducted with the purpose of determining the point at which the incremental cost, effectiveness, or cost-effectiveness of two competing alternatives is neutral.

Time costs. Costs associated with the time a patient spends receiving a medical intervention or receiving medical care.

Time preference. The rate of discounting applied to future events by any given person.

Time trade-off. A method for calculating preference scores in which subjects are asked to condense the quantity of life with a particular disease to achieve perfect health.

Tornado analysis. *See* Sensitivity analysis, tornado.

Triangular distribution. An artificial probability distribution in which the most likely value of a variable is assigned the highest probability of occurring and the lowest and highest plausible value are assigned a probability of 0. All values in between are linearly interpolated.

Two-way sensitivity analysis. *See* Sensitivity analysis, two-way.

Variable costs. Costs that change when a health intervention is applied.

REFERENCES

Advisory Committee on Immunization Practices. "Prevention and Control of Influenza: Recommendations of the Advisory Committee on Immunization Practices (ACIP)." *Morbidity and Mortality Weekly Report,* 2004, *53,* 1–40.

Anderson, R. N. "Method for Constructing Complete Annual U.S. Life Tables." *Vital Health Statistics 2,* 1999, *47,* 1–20.

Attaran, A., and Sachs, J. "Defining and Refining International Donor Support for Combating the AIDS Pandemic." *Lancet,* 2001, *357,* 57–61.

Barendregt, J. J., Bonneux, L., and van der Mass, P. J. "The Health Care Costs of Smoking." *New England Journal of Medicine,* 1997, *337,* 1052–1057.

Berenson, A. "A Cancer Drug Shows Promise, at a Price That Many Can't Pay." *New York Times,* Feb. 15, 2006, p. C1.

Bridges, C. B., and others. "Effectiveness and Cost-Benefit of Influenza Vaccination of Healthy Working Adults." *Journal of the American Medical Association,* 2000, *284,* 1655–1663.

Canadian Task Force on the Periodic Health Examination. "The Periodic Health Examination." *Canadian Medical Association Journal,* 1979, *121,* 1193–1254.

Chrischilles, E. A., and Scholz, D. A. "Dollars and Sense: A Practical Guide to Cost-Analysis for Hospital Epidemiology and Infection Control." *Clinical Performance and Quality Health Care,* 1999, *7*(2), 107–111.

Clissold, S. P., and Heel, R. C. "Topical Minoxidil: A Preliminary Review of Its Pharmacodynamic Properties and Therapeutic Efficacy in Alopecia Areata and Alopecia Androgenetica." *Drugs,* 1987, *33*(2), 107–122.

Dawber, T. R., Kannel, W. E., and Lyell, L. P. "Epidemiological Approaches to Heart Disease: The Framingham Study." *American Journal of Public Health,* 1951, *41,* 279.

de Andrade, H. R., and others. "Chills, Cough and Fever: To Be or Not to Be Influenza." Abstracts P2–79 from Options for the Control of Influenza IV, Hersonissos, Crete, Greece, Sept. 2000.

Doll, R., and Hill, A. B. "Lung Cancer and Other Causes of Death in Relation to Smoking: A Second Report on the Mortality of British Doctors." *British Medical Journal,* 1956, *2,* 1071–1081.

Drug Topics Red Book. Montvale, N.J.: Medical Economics Co., 2006.

Drummond, M. F., O'Brien, B. O., Stoddart, G. L., and Torrance, G. W. *Methods for the Economic Evaluation of Health Care Programmes.* (3rd ed.) New York: Oxford University Press, 2005.

"Epidemics and Economics." *Economist,* Apr. 10, 2003.

Erickson, P., Wilson, R., and Shannon, I. "Years of Healthy Life." *Statistical Notes,* 1995, *7,* 1–16.

EuroQol Group. "EuroQol: A New Facility for the Measurement of Health-Related Quality of Life." *Health Policy,* 1990, *16,* 199–208.

Fahs, M. C., Mandelblatt, J., Schechter, C., and Muller, C. "Cost-Effectiveness of Cervical Cancer Screening for the Elderly." *Annals of Internal Medicine,* 1992, *117,* 520–527.

Farmer, P. *The Pathologies of Power.* Berkeley: University of California Press, 2004.

Fisher, M. J. "Better Living Through the Placebo Effect." *Atlantic Monthly,* Oct. 2000. Retrieved Jan. 2007 from http://profiles.nlm.nih.gov/MM/B/B/R/P/_/mmbbrp.pdf.

Gold, M. R., Franks, P., McCoy, K. I., and Fryback, D. G. "Toward Consistency in Cost-Utility Analyses: Using National Measures to Create Condition-Specific Values." *Medical Care,* 1998, *36,* 778–792.

Gold, M. R., and Muennig, P. "Measure Dependent Variation in Burden of Disease Estimates." *Medical Care,* 2002, *40,* 260–266.

Gold, M. R., Siegel, J. E., Russell, L. B., and Weinstein, M. C. (eds.). *Cost-Effectiveness in Health and Medicine.* New York: Oxford University Press, 1996.

Gotzshe, P. C., and Olsen, O. "Is Screening for Breast Cancer with Mammography Justifiable?" *Lancet,* 2000, *355,* 129–134.

Gyrd-Hansen, D. "Willingness to Pay for a QALY: Theoretical and Methodological Issues." *Pharmacoeconomics,* 2005, *23*(5), 423–432.

Haddix, A. C., Teutsch, S. M., Shaffer, P. A., and Dunet, D. O. *Prevention Effectiveness: A Guide to Decision Analysis and Economic Evaluation.* New York: Oxford University Press, 1996.

Healthcare Cost and Utilization Project, 2006. Retrieved Feb. 23, 2007, from http://hcupnet.ahrq.gov/.

Hirth, R. A., and others. "Willingness to Pay for a Quality-Adjusted Life Year: In Search of a Standard." *Medical Decision Making,* 2000, *20,* 332–32.

Hoyert, D. L., Kung, H. C., and Smith, B. L. "Deaths: Final Data for 2003." *National Vital Statistics Report,* 2005, *53,* 1–48.

Jamison, D. T., Mosley, W. H., Measham, A. R., and Bobadilla, J. L. *Disease Control Priorities in Developing Countries.* New York: Oxford University Press, 1993.

Jeckel, J. F., Elmore, J. G., and Katz, D. L. *Epidemiology, Biostatistics, and Preventive Medicine.* Philadelphia: Saunders, 1996.

Kaplan, R. M., and Anderson, J. P. "A General Health Policy Model: Update and Applications." *Health Services Research,* 1988, *23,* 203–235.

Keech, M., Scott, A. H., and Ryan, P. J. "The Impact of Influenza and Influenza-Like Illness on Productivity and Healthcare Resource Utilization in a Working Population." *Occupational Medicine,* 1998, *48,* 85–90.

Kendal, A. P., Pereria, M. S., and Skehel, J. I. "Concepts and Procedures for Laboratory-Based Influenza Surveillance." Paper presented at the World Health Organization, Geneva, Switzerland, 1982.

Kolata, G. "Medical Fees Are Often Higher for Patients Without Insurance." *New York Times,* Apr. 2, 2001, p. A1.

Lasky, T., and others. "The Guillain-Barré Syndrome and the 1992–1993 and 1993–1994 Influenza Epidemics." *New England Journal of Medicine,* 1998, *339,* 1797–1802.

Lubetkin, E., Jia, H., Franks, P., and Gold, M. R. "Relationship Among Sociodemographic Factors, Clinical Conditions, and Health-Related Quality of Life: Examining the EQ-5D in the U.S. General Population." *Quality of Life Research,* 2005, *12,* 1–10.

Mauskopf, J., Rutten, F., and Schonfeld, W. "Cost-Effectiveness League Tables: Valuable Guidance for Decision Makers?" *Pharmacoeconomics,* 2003, *21,* 991–1000.

Medstat Group. "Medstat Group, 2006." Retrieved Mar. 26, 2007, from http://www.medstat.com.

Meltzer, M. I., Cox, N. J., and Fukuda, K. "The Economic Impact of Pandemic Influenza in the United States: Priorities for Intervention." *Emerging Infectious Disease,* 1999, *5,* 659–671.

Monto, A. S., and others. "Zanamivir in the Prevention of Influenza Among Healthy Adults." *Journal of the American Medical Association,* 1999, *282,* 31–35.

Muennig, P., Franks, P., and Gold, M. "The Cost Effectiveness of Health Insurance." *American Journal of Preventive Medicine,* 2005, *28,* 59–64.

Muennig, P., and Gold, M. R. "Using the Years of Healthy Life Measure to Calculate Quality Adjusted Life Years." *American Journal of Preventive Medicine,* 2001, *20,* 12–17.

Muennig, P. A., and Khan, K. "Cost-Effectiveness of Vaccination Versus Treatment of Influenza in Healthy Adolescents and Adults." *Clinical Infectious Disease,* 2001, *33,* 1879–1885.

Muennig, P., Pallin, D., Sell, R., and Chan, M. S. "The Cost Effectiveness of Strategies for the Treatment of Intestinal Parasites in Immigrants." *New England Journal of Medicine,* 1999, *340,* 773–779.

Muennig, P., and Woolf, S. "The Cost-Effectiveness of Education as a Health Intervention: An Analysis of the Health and Economic Benefits of Reducing the Size of Classes." *American Journal of Public Health,* 2007, *97.*

Muennig, P., and others. "The Income-Associated Burden of Disease in the United States." *Social Science and Medicine,* 2005, *61,* 2018–26.

Murray, C.L.J., and Lopez, A. D. *The Global Burden of Disease: A Comprehensive Assessment of Mortality and Disability from Disease, Injury and Risk Factors in 1990 and Projected to 2020.* Cambridge, Mass.: Harvard University Press, 1996.

National Center for Health Statistics. *Healthy People 2000 Review, 1998–99.* Hyattsville, Md.: Public Health Service, 1999.

National Center for Health Statistics. *Health and Aging Chartbook. Health, United States, 2005.* Hyattsville, Md.: National Center for Health Statistics, 2005.

National Center for Health Statistics. *National Health Interview Survey.* 2006a. Retrieved Mar. 26, 2007, from http://www.cdc.gov/nchs.

National Center for Health Statistics. National Health and Nutrition Examination Survey. 2006b. Retrieved Mar. 26, 2007, from http://www.cdc.gov/nchs/nhanes.htm.

Neumann, P. J., Rosen, A. B., and Weinstein, M. C. "Medicare and Cost-Effectiveness Analysis." *New England Journal of Medicine,* 2005, *355,* 1516–1522.

Neuzil, K. M., Reed, G. W., Mitchel, E. F., and Griffin, M. R. "Influenza-Associated Morbidity and Mortality in Young and Middle-Aged Women." *Journal of the American Medical Association,* 1999, *281,* 901–907.

Nichol, K. L., Margolis, K. L., Wuorenma, J., and Von Sternberg, T. "The Efficacy and Cost-Effectiveness of Vaccination Against Influenza Among Elderly Persons Living in the Community." *New England Journal of Medicine,* 1994, *331,* 778–784.

Olsen, M., and Bailey, M. J. "Positive Time Preference." *Journal of Political Economy,* 1981, *89,* 1–24.

Oregon Health Services Commission. "Oregon Medicaid Priority Setting Project." Portland: Oregon State Government, 1991.

Oregon Office for Health Policy and Research. "Oregon Health Plan." May 2001. Retrieved Mar. 26, 2007, from http://www.ohppr.state.or.us/.

Owings, M. F., and Lawrence, L. "Detailed Diagnoses and Procedures. National Hospital Discharge Survey, 1997. National Center for Health Statistics." *Vital Health Statistics,* 1999, *13,* 1–163.

Petersen, M. "Lifting the Curtain on the Real Costs of Making AIDS Drugs." *New York Times,* Apr. 24, 2001, p. C1.

Rabin, R., and de Charro, F. "EQ-5D: A Measure of Health Status from the EuroQol Group." *Annals of Medicine,* 2001, *33,* 337–343.

Schaller, D. R., and Olson, B. H. "A Food Industry Perspective on Folic Acid Fortification." *Journal of Nutrition,* 1996, *126,* 761S–764S.

Schappert, S. M., and Nelson, C. "National Ambulatory Medical Care Survey, 1995–96." *Vital Health Statistics,* 1999, *13,* i-vi, 1–122.

Secker-Walker, R. H., and others. "Screening for Breast Cancer: Time in Travel and Out-of-Pocket Expenses." *Journal of the National Cancer Institute,* 1999, *91,* 702–708.

Shaw, J. W., Johnson, J. A., and Coons, S. J. "U.S. Valuation of the EQ-5D Health States: Development and Testing of the D1 Valuation Model." *Medical Care,* 2005, *43*(3), 203–220.

Strauss, R. S. "Comparison of Measured and Self-Reported Weight and Height in a Cross-Sectional Sample of Young Adolescents." *International Journal of Obesity and Related Metabolic Disorders,* 1999, *23*(8), 904–908.

Tengs, T. O., and others. "Five Hundred Life-Saving Interventions and Their Cost-Effectiveness." *Risk Analysis,* 1995, *15,* 369–390.

Thelle, D. S., Arnesen, E., and Forde, O. H. "The Tromso Heart Study: Does Coffee Raise Serum Cholesterol?" *New England Journal of Medicine,* 1983, *308,* 1454–1457.

Treanor, J. J., and others. "Efficacy and Safety of the Oral Neuraminidase Inhibitor Oseltamivir in Treating Acute Influenza." *Journal of the American Medical Association,* 2000, *283,* 1016–1024.

Ubel, P. A., DeKay, M. L., Baron, J., and Asch, D. A. "Cost-Effectiveness Analysis in a Setting of Budget Constraints—Is It Equitable?" *New England Journal of Medicine,* 1996, *334,* 1174–1177.

U.S. Bureau of the Census. *Current Population Reports. Money Income in the United States: 1998.* Washington, D.C.: Government Printing Office, 1999.

U.S. Food and Drug Administration. "Food Labeling: Trans Fatty Acids in Nutrition Labeling, Nutrient Content Claims, and Health Claims; Proposed Rule." *Federal Register,* Nov. 17, 1999.

Urgert, R., and others. "Comparison of Effect of Cafetiere and Filtered Coffee on Serum Concentrations of Liver Aminotransferases and Lipids: Six Month Randomised Controlled Trial." *British Medical Journal,* 1996, *313,* 1362–1366.

Wennberg, J., and Gittelsohn, A. "Variations in Medical Care Among Small Areas." *Scientific American,* 1982, *246,* 120–134.

Wilkinson, R. G. "Health, Hierarchy, and Social Anxiety." *Annals of the New York Academy of Science,* 1999, *896,* 48–63.

World Health Organization. "WHO Guide to Cost-Effectiveness Analysis." Geneva: World Health Organization, 2003. Retrieved Mar. 26, 2007, from http://www.who.int/choice/en/.

World Health Organization. *Working Together for Health.* Geneva: World Health Organization, 2006.

Wynn, M., and Wynn, A. "Fortification of Grain Products with Folate: Should Britain Follow the American Example?" *Nutrition and Health,* 1998, *12,* 147–161.

INDEX